P9-CED-091

Trim and Sculpt Your Body in Less Than Six Weeks

BODY EXPRESS
MAKEOVER

MICHAEL GEORGE

A FIRESIDE BOOK
PUBLISHED BY SIMON & SCHUSTER

NEW YORK   LONDON   TORONTO   SYDNEY

FIRESIDE
Rockefeller Center
1230 Avenue of the Americas
New York, NY 10020

Copyright © 2005 by Michael George
All rights reserved,
including the right of reproduction in whole or in part in any form.

FIRESIDE and colophon are registered trademarks of Simon & Schuster, Inc.

For information regarding special discounts for bulk purchases,
please contact Simon & Schuster Special Sales at 1-800-456-6798
or business@simonandschuster.com

Designed by Ruth Lee Mui

Manufactured in the United States of America

2   4   6   8   10   9   7   5   3   1

Library of Congress Cataloging-in-Publication Data

George, Michael, 1948–
Body express makeover : trim and sculpt your body in less than six weeks / Michael George.
    p.   cm.
Includes index.
1. Physical fitness.   2. Nutrition.   3. Exercise.   4. Health.   I. Title.
    RA781.G44   2005
    613.7'1—dc22
    2005041262

ISBN 0-7432-6121-6

This publication contains the opinions and ideas of its author. It is intended to provide helpful and in-formative material on the subjects addressed in the publication. It is sold with the understanding that the author and publisher are not engaged in rendering medical, health, or any other kind of personal professional services in the book. The reader should consult his or her medical, health, or other com-petent professional before adopting any of the suggestions in this book or drawing inferences from it.

The author and publisher specifically disclaim all responsibility for any liability, loss, or risk, per-sonal or otherwise, which is incurred as a consequence, directly or indirectly, of the use and applica-tion of any of the contents of this book.

D E D I C A T I O N

I dedicate this book to my dear friend Lysa Renee Charles who lost her battle with lupus on February 27, 2004. Lysa was not only one of my closest friends, but she was the most positive, happy, selfless person I have ever met in my entire life. She was and still is loved by so many. Lysa and I met in college and quickly came to be good friends not knowing then that our friendship would last until her death. Fourteen years ago Lysa was diagnosed with the catastrophic disease of lupus, which savagely attacks the body's immune system and destroys major vital organs. She went through years of intense pain and suffering and was on dialysis for many of those years awaiting a new kidney, but during this time she was always positive, laughing, and happy. She never wanted anyone to worry about her and she never felt sorry for herself. She just fought for her life with a zeal I've never seen before. The courage she demonstrated was incomprehensible.

Lysa was a very old soul who was touched by the hand of God. I truly believe she was an angel in disguise. Even before she got lupus, Lysa always had a positive attitude and was always your number-one supporter. She was a person who gave you all of herself. She rarely spoke about herself, but always wanted to know about you and how your life was going. She was the most unselfish person on earth. The first time we thought she might not pull through, her parents called me. I went to her house and she was lying on the bed too tired to even talk. She asked me to hold her hand, which I did for hours while she slept and I watched television. The sadness I felt leaving her that night was unimaginable. However, she pulled through that time.

Lysa was only a few days away from having heart surgery to repair her heart from the damage of lupus so she could then have her second kidney transplant—her first kidney had failed due to a misprescribed medication. Then disaster struck. Her heart valve exploded and she died. I, as do all her friends and family, miss having Lysa in our lives. If you were feeling down or blue Lysa would always cheer you up. She was my staunchest supporter when everyone else thought I was crazy for quitting my job as a financial analyst and moving to Los Angeles to pursue my dream. I owe this book to Lysa for never letting me quit on myself and for always helping me to see the bright side of life. I will always be grateful for having Lysa in my life. If there were more people like her this world would be a much better place to live in. Until we meet again, Lysa, I just want to say I did it and I love you.

ACKNOWLEDGMENTS

Being given the opportunity to write this book was a dream come true for me. There are so many people to thank for their support, guidance, and friendship, but none more deserving of my appreciation and gratitude than my good friend Julie Arde. Julie was my rock, my sounding board, and the

person who helped me edit the entire book. She has always supported me in my career, but her efforts on my behalf to make sure this book was the best it could possibly be were nothing less than extraordinary. After a long day at work she would come over to my house and work on my book late into the evening, night after night, without even a grumble. She edited the book on numerous weekends, pushing aside her own tasks. It was she who turned my endless run-on sentences and wordy paragraphs into a succinct structure that was readable. For all of her editorial efforts, her unconditional love, her constant support, her selfless friendship, and her quirky sense of humor that always makes me laugh, I owe Julie an everlasting thank-you from the bottom of my heart. I couldn't have written this book without her.

Thanking everyone for their help and support is such a daunting task because there are so many people to thank for making this book a reality. I want to thank my literary agent, Mike Harriot, for initially contacting me to write this book and Carolyn Sutton for believing in me and purchasing the book on behalf of Simon &

Schuster. I want to thank Cherise Davis, my editor at Simon & Schuster, for being thrust into a difficult situation and really doing an unprecedented job at guiding me through the process of writing this book. I also want to thank her for believing in me as a writer and for all her wonderful suggestions. I also need to thank Marcia Burch, Ellen Silberman, Trina Rice, and everyone else at Simon & Schuster who worked hard to make this book the best it could be.

I owe much thanks to my assistant Alex Smay for always having my back and Dr. Barry Sears for his support, friendship, and for writing the wonderful foreword that he wrote on my behalf. I would like to thank Tom Woods for his continual support as well. I owe many thanks to my photographer, Allison Dyer, and her patience for shooting endless photos over and over again. I am very appreciative of the hard work all my models put in; Gloria Rodriguez, Whitney Padgett, and of course, Julie Arde. I also want to thank all of my clients over the past eighteen years for allowing me to train them and for putting up with my crazy ideas when it came to new exercises and training techniques. I have great appreciation for their trust in me, their support, their friendship, and for giving me the blessed opportunity to be a part of their lives. Every one of my clients has enriched my life and taught me so much about what it means to be a good human.

There is a long list, too long, of numerous associates and peers to thank for all their support and who were always ready to help me in any capacity. I would like to thank Jackie Geller, owner of Nutrifit in Los Angeles, for all her endless guidance and support. I would like to thank all of my numerous yoga and martial arts instructors who taught me the Eastern mind-set, which helps guide my spiritual life. I owe my life, as it is today, to my mentor and spiritual guide, Tony Pace, who is no longer with us. I also owe much gratitude to Tim Eckerman, who gave an eighteen-year-old sopping wet city boy a job as a ski technician in a small mountain resort ski shop. He then proceeded to teach me the meaning of self-respect, responsibility, and what it means to be accountable as an adult. I never did get the chance to thank him for caring and for being instrumental in my decision to attend college. Thank you, Tim, for extending yourself to a young teenager desperate for guidance.

Last, I have to thank my friends and family. I need to thank them for putting up with me when I canceled plans or turned down social events because I needed to write. I respect and appreciate your friendship and your love. I'm sure there are people I have left out, but please know that you are in my heart and your assistance has not been forgotten. Thank you to all who made this book possible and supported me on my journey.

CONTENTS

CONTENTS

FOREWORD

Have you ever wondered what secrets Hollywood stars use to maintain a body composition that most of us only dream about? Or how contestants in shows such as *Extreme Makeover* can change their body shape in a matter of weeks? Well, there is no magic pill or potion, simply the application of smart nutrition and insightful physical training. But you have to have a plan, and Michael George provides exactly that in *Body Express Makeover*.

Your goal is to have good body composition and the wellness that goes with it in the shortest possible amount of time, yet keep it for the longest period of time. That means having a strategy that you can stick with for a lifetime. These are key concepts in Michael's book. You have to eat, so you might as well eat intelligently so that you burn incoming calories as fuel, as opposed to storing them as fat. To do so, you have to keep your hormones, especially insulin, within a tight zone throughout the day. It's not that difficult if you follow Michael's tips.

Then there is exercise. Time is the enemy. Michael provides a revolutionary approach to burning the maximum number of calories in the smallest amount of time. It's a disciplined approach, but once you understand the concepts, there becomes no excuse for lack of exercise. As you might expect, there is no one magical type of exercise, simply a requirement to build a "three-legged stool" consisting of endurance, strength, and flexibility.

Nutrition and exercise remain the keys to not only a better body, but, more important, a lifetime of wellness. If those are your goals, reading and practicing the concepts in this book are the primary "drugs" you will need.

—Dr. Barry Sears, author of *The Zone*

AUTHOR'S NOTE

Are you ready to change your life? Are you ready to become the you you have always dreamed of being? Are you ready to lose unwanted pounds quickly? If you are ready to make this change, this book and the programs contained in it will change your body and your lifestyle in ways you can't imagine.

My name is Michael George. My passion is to help transform as many lives as I can in this lifetime, and that's exactly what I have been doing for the past twenty years. I have developed a revolutionary training system with a proven eating strategy that will help you drop excess body fat, tone and sculpt your muscles, and build lean muscle mass with a nutritional structure that you can adhere to for life without ever having to go hungry or feel deprived.

For twenty years I have been training actors, models, dancers, singers, executives, and housewives to help them achieve their health and fitness goals. Clients come to me for many reasons and in various stages of change. I have helped some clients lose fifty to eighty pounds, brides-to-be lose those last ten pounds for that special day, and numerous actors and models get into tip-top shape fast for that big movie or photo shoot. It doesn't matter what your goal is, the Body Express Makeover will educate you and enlighten you on how to get fit and live a healthy lifestyle. The exercise programs and nutritional guidelines contained in this book are designed to change your body fast, make no

mistake about that; but throughout this process you should constantly envision what living a healthy lifestyle looks and feels like for you. Feel how empowered you would be by making the choice to exercise and eat healthfully for the rest of your life.

I want you to know that each and every one of you has the courage, strength, patience, and tenacity to succeed. All you have to do is look deep into your heart for these qualities, which will support your every step. In the boxing ring, it's not the fighter with the best technical skills or the hardest punch, or even the better athlete, who wins; it's the fighter who has heart and who won't let anything stand in his way. It's the fighter who will do whatever it takes to succeed, so that when the final bell rings, his hand is the one raised in victory.

I'm not going to ignore the fact that many of you have tried to lose weight, tone up, or get fit and have come up short or empty-handed. I understand that frustration and will address obstacles and self-defeating behavior throughout this book. However, success is built upon failure after failure. In order to succeed at anything in life, you have to embrace failure in order to learn the valuable lessons along the way. You need to learn what to do and what not to do. Success is all about being present in the moment. Being present is when we realize that we are already perfect as we are. We are whole and unique individuals right now. Success is about understanding that the past is the past and has nothing to do with the present or future except for the power you give to it.

Here is my promise to you: If you give me your trust . . . if you make the commitment necessary to succeed and believe that you can . . . if you give this process your heart . . . you will succeed in whatever goals you are striving to attain.

The Body Express Makeover will provide you with the knowledge, training strategy, and nutritional guidance that will empower you and propel you to the winner's circle in the fastest time possible. How can I make such outlandish claims? Because I have seen these kinds of success stories every day for the past twenty years. I will not lie to you: it will take effort on your part. But the effort you put into this program will come back a hundredfold and will provide you with a lifelong way of exercising and healthy eating patterns that will support one another and support living a healthy lifestyle.

With the Body Express Makeover, you will have the body you've always dreamed of, and you will be proud of that fact.

This is my promise to you.

Now it is time for you.

INTRODUCTION

There is a reason you are reading this book. Maybe you are frustrated that you just can't lose those last ten pounds. Maybe you want to really sculpt your body but haven't been successful on your own. Maybe you just need a time-efficient exercise regime. Or maybe you just need a new challenge, something different. Whatever your goals, the Body Express Makeover will help you attain them. It all starts with the stage of change you are in and where your commitment level stands right now. How important is changing your body and your life?

The Body Express Makeover is a very effective shortcut to help you reach your fitness goals in the shortest amount of time. Here's how it works. A proven nutritional strategy will help to raise your metabolism and support your natural fat-burning functions to operate at their highest levels. Aided by a very realistic and consistent aerobic activity schedule, that layer of fat now covering your muscles will melt away. My unique 2-in-1 Body Express Strength Training exercises will then tone and shape every muscle in your body, completing your total body makeover. But this isn't the best part. The best part is that you can achieve this makeover in just a few short weeks—without spending hours in the gym every day. That's the Body Express Makeover!

The Body Express exercise programs are an extension of my own personal evolution as an athlete and as a personal trainer. During this evolution I trained in boxing and martial arts, and became a yoga practitioner, while consistently studying new exercise modalities such as Pilates, core strengthening, body structure, functional training, and plyometrics. All of these training disciplines are incorporated into the Body Express Makeover exercise programs.

Sports and exercise became the road map to change my body but soon became my passion in life. My participation in sports and exercise created a desire in me to engage in new activities such as mountain biking, snow skiing and waterskiing, tennis, and golf, which in turn provided me a very active and healthy lifestyle. After being introduced to Eastern disciplines such as martial arts and yoga, I immediately gravitated to their mind/body philosophies. While disciplines such as yoga became a method for me to quiet my inner self and reduce stress, they also provided balance in my workout regimen and increased flexibility. Additionally, martial arts and boxing helped me release pent-up emotions and challenged me to learn new skills such as self-defense.

With my truly diverse background in physical fitness, including team sports, amateur bodybuilding, martial arts, and yoga, it was only natural for me to begin teaching. I decided to combine these techniques and training methods, become multicertified, and begin a career as a personal trainer. I wanted to help others achieve the same dramatic transformation that I had. I began extensive study and research into nutrition, human performance, and the various innate mechanisms the human body uses to regulate its metabolism and store and lose body fat. I combined these principles and created a comprehensive program for a total body transformation. The Body Express Makeover is a revolutionary and modern approach to correct the imbalances in your life. When you correct the imbalances in your life, you will quickly transform your body.

Lack of time is the number one obstacle when it comes to getting fit and living a healthy lifestyle. In this country, time is one of the great imbalances many of us are challenged by each day. Simply put, we are overwhelmed. Technology has brought us the answering machine, fax, mobile phone, and e-mail. In today's society, it is commonplace for people to check voice mails and e-mails throughout each day. As if that wasn't enough, you then have to open your mailbox and sort through the junk mail and bills. To pay those bills, most of us are working ten hours a week more than we did a decade ago, and many American workers are being forced to do the work of two or three employees due to downsizing. Because we are working more hours, we are also sitting for longer periods of time and getting less daily activity, which promotes weight gain and muscular dysfunc-

tion. Although technology has improved our efficiency and made our lives easier in numerous ways, it has also made us fatter and increased our chances of injuring ourselves. Today, 80 percent of our population has some form of back pain due to muscular dysfunction or being overweight.

There are also family responsibilities (see where the priorities are upside down?) as well as social responsibilities and interaction. After all that, how much time do you have for yourself? You need time to work, eat, relax, and play with your children or help them with homework. When is there time to take care of yourself? Our lives look like a complicated juggling act, and we have a lot of balls in the air. The point is this: you are the juggler. If you do not take care of yourself first and foremost, everything—*and I mean everything*—will suffer, as you may already have discovered.

Lack of time is also one of the great excuses. You may be saying to yourself, "I just don't have the time to fit exercise into my life." In fact, if you don't take the time to correct the imbalances in your life, you won't have much more time. Let me reiterate: time will essentially run out for you. If you feel that you don't have enough time in your life, let me suggest that TIME is precisely what is out of balance in your life. It's time to stop being a slave to the clock and start taking control of your life and your responsibilities.

For most of my celebrity clients, time is at a premium, what with reading scripts, attending events, promoting new films, traveling to and from locations, and then, of course, actually acting. This meant that I needed to find a way to get them into shape for their film or modeling projects fast. I needed to find a way to work all their muscle groups harder and faster so that results could be seen in weeks as opposed to months. I began to experiment by combining various exercises. I used all the knowledge and training techniques I had acquired over the previous twenty years of training both my clients and myself. I began to think "out of the box." I kept trying new exercises and asking myself, "What if?" The result was the methodology I designed to work every muscle and muscle group in just ten minutes.

Most traditional strength training regimes require a lot of time in the gym. When they are strength training, most people work one muscle group at a time or go from machine to machine, maybe spending several minutes working one particular muscle group and resting in between sets. Training this way just isn't efficient enough. It takes too long to get through an entire workout, not to mention the fact that there really is no cardiovascular component to such a workout. I began asking myself, "Why can't I work two or more muscle groups at the same time?" I started to mix yoga postures and martial arts stances and kicks with strength training exercises. I blended Pilates techniques and core training with strength training exercises. I reduced the rest time in between sets to keep my clients' heart rate up, in an effort to build endurance and burn more calories. The result was the 2-in-1 Body Express training system, a blend of East and West, of strength and stamina. As you work multiple muscle groups simultaneously, with very little rest in between sets, your heart rate remains elevated, increasing the intensity of the workout. The result: you burn more calories in a shorter amount of time and

strengthen your cardiovascular system, all within a total body workout time of only ten minutes. In short, you are actually doing aerobic training and strength training simultaneously.

This new exercise system eventually became the core of my strength training regimens with all of my clients. Even I found these shorter workouts both challenging and effective. I added new exercises to this regimen and created exercises to stretch the workout to twenty minutes and then to thirty minutes. I was soon using these unique ten-, twenty-, and thirty-minute 2-in-1 workouts in my personal training practice. My clients became walking billboards, advertisements for how effective my new system was at getting fast results.

Soon Hollywood clients began calling my method *the* hot new workout." It seemed that this particular methodology was tailor-made to meet their needs. Without exception, all of them had a very short time to get into shape or, at a minimum, maintain their current physique. A mildly overweight actress needed to look more like Xena, the Warrior Princess. A rather demure woman needed to be believable as an active, forceful army captain. Another, after the birth of her third child, needed to go from a size 12 to a size 4 in three months, because half of a movie that had been filmed two years before had to be reshot. While all the actors and actresses I work with vary in age and physical fitness, all of them always need to look their best quickly—and that is precisely what you want to do too.

I will honestly tell you that the Body Express strength training system works! It will help you achieve a better body and a healthier life *fast.* In the process, you will reduce your stress levels, become more present, and as a result, be more efficient and creative in your workplace. You will see your relationships with your friends and family improve dramatically because you will have a more positive outlook on life and your tolerance of others' shortcomings will be increased due to this shift in attitude. All of these improvements will add up to your being healthier, happier, and more empowered.

Over time, you will increase your immune capacity and improve your heart function. You will greatly reduce your chance of developing debilitating diseases such as diabetes, stroke, Parkinson's, heart attack, and many forms of cancer. If you get on board the Body Express Makeover, you will be less likely to experience feelings of depression. If you stay on board long enough, you will increase your chances of being mentally and physically active when you celebrate your hundredth birthday.

If you get on board the Body Express, you can become the YOU you always wanted to be. Dreams are meant to come true if you just believe in them wholeheartedly. That is my promise to you.

BODY EXPRESS
MAKEOVER

CHAPTER ONE

GET ON BOARD

The Body Express Makeover is designed to help you change your body and get the results you are looking for effectively and efficiently. It is a superfast, revolutionary training system designed to trim, shape, and sculpt your body into the best that it can possibly be. But the best part of this revolu-

tionary training system is not the results you will see when you look in the mirror; the best part is that by changing your body, you will also transform your level of self-esteem and self-confidence and become more effective and empowered in your life as a whole.

I have an extremely high success rate when it comes to helping my clients achieve their fitness goals—first, because I motivate and encourage them to make a very strong commitment to the process right out of the gate, and second, because I persuade them not to focus on losing weight as their primary goal but to focus on a whole host of other results they will experience throughout the process of achieving their weight loss goals.

Constantly focusing on simply losing weight is a setup for failure, because no matter how fast you lose weight, it will never be fast enough, and you risk setting yourself up for all the negative self-talk that comes with feeling discouraged. Also, by focusing only on how fast the extra body fat is coming off, you miss the big picture of what consistent exercise and a healthful diet will bring to your life as a whole. So I

urge you to do exactly what I tell my clients to do: focus on the big picture. I know that you most likely want to lose a certain amount of body fat, and you will if you follow the Body Express Makeover training system. But I want you to focus on how much better you feel rather than how you look. I promise you that this way of approaching your new exercise regime will be much more motivating over the long haul and will dramatically increase your success rate.

Clients come to me in various stages of change. One of the secrets of success is knowing what stage of change you are in. Honoring that stage of change and knowing how committed you are to making lasting change is vital. There is an old saying that you can lead a horse to water, but you can't make it drink. It's true. As your coach, I will do everything in my power to educate you and guide you to your ultimate goal, but in the end it is not me on the field, the track, or the court playing the game; it's you. How badly you want a new body and lifestyle will determine your success.

The focus of this chapter is to motivate you to make the choice to go from contemplation to action. To do so, I feel it is important to lay out some very dismal statistics that will, I hope, open your eyes to some trends that are jeopardizing our country's well-being as a whole.

- 64.5 percent (approximately two thirds of the U.S. population, about 127 million people) of Americans are overweight and 30 percent clinically obese. These numbers have doubled since 1980 and increased by 10 percent in the last four years. The estimated number of premature deaths caused by obesity is 300,000 annually. Obesity ranks second after smoking as a preventable cause of death.
- According to the National Center of Chronic Disease Prevention and Health Promotion, from 1980 to 2002 the number of Americans with diabetes more than doubled from 5.8 million to 13.3 million.
- Americans spend $30 billion every year trying to control or lose weight.
- In 1970, the total American expenditure on fast food was $6 billion; in 2000, that figure was $110 billion.
- Cancer is the number two killer in America and is responsible for one of every four deaths in America. More than 1,500 people die every day from cancer. U.S. women have a 1 in 10 chance of developing cancer. Regular exercise can reduce the risk of cancer by at least 50 percent.
- Heart disease and stroke are the first and third leading causes of death in the U.S. and account for 40 percent of all deaths, approximately one death every 33 seconds.

Are those not startling statistics? Do they motivate you to make a change? There are six stages you will go through to complete the change that you desire (see box). And congratulations! By buying and reading this book, you have conquered and moved past the first stage of change—precontemplation.

The Body Express Makeover is designed specifically to address each phase of change. In

---

THE SIX STAGES OF CHANGE

1. **PRECONTEMPLATION:** You can't see any problem, have no intention of changing your behavior, you deny having a problem, and you don't want to change yourself, only the people around you.
2. **CONTEMPLATION:** You have a desire to stop feeling so stuck. You acknowledge that there is a problem, struggle to understand it, and begin to think seriously about changing it. You can visualize the destination and even how to get there, but you're not ready to go yet and still far from taking action.
3. **PREPARATION:** You plan to take action within the month and are making the final adjustments before beginning to change your behaviors—cutting short the preparation stage, i.e., quitting cold turkey, lowers your chance of success.
4. **ACTION:** You modify your behavior and your environment. This is the busiest period and requires the greatest commitment of time and energy.
5. **MAINTENANCE:** You work to consolidate the gains you've attained and struggle to prevent relapses. Maintenance is a tremendous challenge that requires a strong, long-term commitment.
6. **TERMINATION:** This is your ultimate goal. You will no longer be tempted by bad behavior and you will have the confidence of being able to cope without fear of relapses.

chapter 1, I will motivate you to contemplate the change that lies ahead. In chapter 2, we will obliterate the preparation stage by solidifying your commitment to making the change by utilizing a journal and a calendar. I will also answer many questions you may have about the Body Express training system and discuss all the areas of your life that will be improved in the process of transforming your body. In chapter 3, we will begin to prepare a clear, focused course of action. In the remaining chapters, I will propel you into action by teaching you how to eat healthfully and the importance of both aerobic and resistance exercise. Then I will guide you through the strength and stretching routines, which will transform your body and your lifestyle, ending with the maintenance phase of this training system, which is a program you can follow for the rest of your life. You will learn how to maintain your transformation and reach your ultimate goal—no matter how great that goal is.

This training system absolutely works. If you follow my suggestions and the programs in this book, you will change your body and, in the process, your life. I can make such statements because I have seen the results with my own eyes with hundreds of my own clients. I say this with confidence because you see these results with your own eyes when you go to a movie or turn on the television. I can promise you that you will change your body and your life because the Body Express training system has changed my clients' bodies and lives and continues to do so every day.

The Body Express Makeover offers something for everyone. If you do not exercise or have not done so for some time, you may feel challenged at first. The strength training routines may be a little difficult in the beginning, but you will catch on quickly and see results much faster than with any other programs you may have tried. If you already exercise regularly, these programs will represent an epiphany of method and time efficiency and motivate you to achieve greater levels of physical fitness in addition to a more sculpted body. Those of you who are already extreme athletes will find this new method of training challenging and motivating due to the revolutionary new exercises, which will rejuvenate your workouts. Regardless of your age, your level of fitness, or how dramatically you would like to change your body, the Body Express Makeover programs will change the way you exercise forever.

These programs are my calling. They are my passion. The longer I am in the fitness industry, the more passionate I become. What drives me is the process. It is the process you are embarking on right now. It is the process of transforming your body and, by doing so, transforming your life. I have written this book to guide you through what I refer to as healthy lifestyle transformation.

The Body Express Makeover is not like dipping your toes into a pool to test the water temperature. It is about jumping into the deep end with the understanding that you have the innate ability to swim and take control of your health. My programs are all about time. I've designed the most time-efficient body transformation system for one purpose: to save you precious time. I have designed this training system to help you achieve all of your fitness goals. But there's a catch: I can't achieve them for you. You will have to do the work. If I could do it for you,

I gladly would, but it just doesn't work that way. I can, however, provide you with the tools, knowledge, and training techniques you will need and educate you on how to incorporate this information into a very simple plan of action.

The key to achieving all your fitness goals is your desire to change your current situation. There are two things in life that motivate us: pleasure and pain. We naturally seek pleasure and try to avoid pain. When the pain becomes too great, it is time to take action. It is now time to reduce the pain and increase the pleasure in your life. Clients come to me because they are unhappy with their body and ready to make a change. Even though it may not be in the forefront of their mind, there is a degree of pain in the form of frustration that motivated them to pick up the phone and call me. It is important to look at this closely and honestly. You really have to want the change you are about to create. You must want this for yourself—not for anyone else. You must want it more than anything. It must become a top priority in your life.

Changing your body can be a real head trip. Many of you may have done the roller-coaster ride with your weight throughout most of your life. This success/failure pattern can create many deep and personal issues surrounding changing your body and your appearance. We lug so much emotional baggage with us when we diet or begin an exercise program that our "stuff" weighs on us in the back of our minds. I'm asking you to check your emotional baggage at the door. You are embarking on a new approach to changing your body with a revolutionary training system that has an extremely high success rate. Remember, the past is the past. It has nothing to do with the present or the future except the power you give it.

It does not matter what kind of physical condition you are in right now or how great the physical transformation you would like to achieve. The Body Express Makeover can take you to whatever destination you choose. You can and will change the way you look, the way you feel, and the way you feel about yourself. You deserve to feel fantastic about yourself and your life. Life is too short to be unhappy about your appearance. Trust me, I know. My intention is to take you to that place so when you look in the mirror you love who and what is being reflected back at you.

When I work with clients, much of my work involves discovering the complex pieces of their puzzle and coaching them through the assembly process. As a transformation coach, my job begins with getting into my clients' heads, finding out what is going on inside, and then planting some seeds that will bear fruit for them. I must determine what prevents them from achieving their health and wellness goals. In short, I unearth self-defeating patterns or negative lifestyle habits that short-circuit my clients' ability to achieve their ultimate goals. Once I determine their shortcomings and self-defeating behaviors, I make my clients aware of them so that they can work to overcome them. You are eminently capable of discovering these stopping points for yourself, and in this chapter I will provide you with some suggestions to help you navigate around them.

Perhaps you will read some things in this chapter that will resonate with you. If you read something that evokes a negative emotional response, that's okay, just take notice. I want you to pay attention to any emotional response, whether it be anger, irritation, or even sadness. The most important and profound relationship in life is the relationship you have with yourself. The quickest and most tangible way to improve that relationship is through the physical. When you consciously work to improve your physical being (your body), you directly improve your intellectual, emotional, and spiritual capacity and potential. While this work can become your own personal shortcut toward personal growth, it is definitely the most time-efficient method of elevating and enhancing your relationship with yourself. By nurturing this relationship, you will most certainly enhance your relationship with the world around you.

I grew up in a household of immigrants. My parents came of age in a different world, one that was filled with the horrors of war and the famine left in the wake of that war. When they came to a land of prosperity and abundance, they overcompensated for having had to go without for all those years. Like all good parents, mine wanted me to have everything that they hadn't had as children. As a result, our lives centered on the dinner table, and happiness was defined by heavy, fat-laden foods in large quantities. Because my parents literally knew what it was like to starve, nothing was wasted, and not eating all your food was unacceptable. As you can probably guess, I became more overweight with each passing year. By the time I entered grade school, I was clinically obese.

My parents moved often, and in each new school and each new city, I was the new kid . . . the fat kid . . . the kid who didn't belong . . . the kid who couldn't fit in. Being overweight really damaged my level of self-worth. I was with-drawn and shy. I had difficulty reaching out to people. I lacked the confidence to build friend-ships, to become involved, and to excel in any-thing that might draw more attention to myself. I was keenly aware of and sensitive to the way people perceived me. I was truly embarrassed about the way I looked and ashamed of my body. The more shame I felt, the deeper I with-drew into myself. Being overweight was a painful experience, and I desperately wished I could just be invisible. It is this connection with the pain of being overweight that I have in com-mon with many of my clients and many of you. It is why I understand your need to change your body fast.

But let's get back to the story. Another city, another school . . . The chip on my shoulder was ten times bigger than the number on the scale. I immediately gravitated toward others like myself—definitely the wrong crowd. Trou-ble followed, and wherever it went, I wanted to be in the middle of it. I finally found a crowd that accepted me, and I did everything I could to get their approval. When I was a teenager, drugs and petty crimes were no strangers to me. As I sunk deeper and deeper, I began to get into trouble with the law. I seemed to be in a vicious cycle. I truly believe that the cycle began with my being overweight: I didn't like myself, and I used negative attention to gain affection. I be-came someone I was not, and on some level, I hated myself all the more for doing that to my-self. Self-loathing and self-destructive behavior perpetuated themselves into a cycle of negativity that permeated my entire being.

Since the moment I became aware that I was different and that I was obese, I fantasized about looking different. I don't know if you will be able to relate to this, but I didn't just want to look different—I wanted to become another person. If you are old enough to remember him, Charles Atlas was a revered pioneer of bodybuilding. His mythically muscle-popping physique was the gold standard to which generations of men aspired. Conjure up that image, and I was further away from that svelte physique than one could ever dream. For some reason, I identified with that mental image and got hooked on the dream of looking something— anything—like that ideal. I wanted to look the exact opposite of my reflection in the mirror. I don't know why, but somehow I ordered the Charles Atlas Weight Training System. That event changed my life forever. In fact, it probably saved it.

I yearned to look like and become a different person. It was my highest aspiration and my greatest dream. The dream was delivered to me at the age of sixteen in the form of a book much like this one: *The Charles Atlas 12-Week Training System.* It did not come with any equipment, just weight-training programs. Undaunted, I dived into the book. I then tore up some bricks around my mother's garden and taped them to a wooden baseball bat to use as a barbell. I began using Charles Atlas's program religiously, changed my diet, and began jogging daily. Very quickly, my life began to change in ways I could not have imagined.

I began to feel differently about myself. At the time it wasn't tangible or even something that I was consciously aware of, but in retrospect I now recognize that I simply felt more self-confident and empowered. For perhaps the first time in my life, I felt hopeful instead of hopeless. That small dose of self-esteem was like a

"time-release capsule" that began to change my life. My attitude had completely changed. I started doing better in school, applying effort to everything I did. For the first time in my life, I took pride in my schoolwork, in the way in which I expressed myself, and in my appearance.

After just a few months, there were no more bricks left around my mother's garden. My parents were so relieved and thankful that I had gravitated toward something positive that my father purchased an actual set of free weights and a weight bench for me. And in just six short months, I lost more than fifty pounds and much of my old self. People started to notice the changes to my body. I started getting attention from girls for the first time. I began living life on a straight-and-narrow path, raised my grade point average, and began making friends with new people who had direction. I had always been involved with organized sports, but I began to really excel. I enjoyed each sport with a renewed zeal because I was stronger, more confident, and a much better athlete. Sports became my first love. Training became my passion, and I worked harder and harder, became fitter and fitter. One activity led to many other activities, such as wrestling, football, and tennis.

I turned my life around in a very short amount of time, and you can too. I was not superhuman or any different from you except for the fact that I was extremely motivated to make drastic changes in my life. I owe it all to the benefits derived from exercise and sports. Not only did I radically transform my physical appearance, but I also underwent an equally valuable overhaul of my self-esteem. What really hooked me was that exercise (truly, any form of exercise) improved how I felt about myself. I began to appreciate and treasure my life in ways I had never dreamed of. After exercising, I felt positive, hopeful, energized, and—perhaps for the first time in a long time—happy.

My overall disposition changed from dark and dour to excited, eager, and engaged. Rather than feeling "apart," I became closer to my family and my peers and felt more comfortable in my own skin and in the world. I noticed my level of ambition soar. Through exercise and sports, I learned self-discipline. By taking control of my body, I had real and tangible proof that I could take control of my life. By taking control of my life, I discovered that I had the power to improve the world around me. Because of the empowerment I experienced through exercise, I gained the courage to better my surroundings, my relationships, and now my community. It is this evolution that drove me to write this book.

Whether you are nineteen or ninety, the Body Express Makeover will take you on a very similar journey and enable you to have a life-changing experience. The real secret is that the inner feelings of increased self-worth, self-empowerment, and self-love are the real goals of your workouts. Why? Because it is these qualities that will motivate you to make eating healthfully and exercising a part of your lifestyle and give you the body you've always dreamed of having. You will understand what I'm taking about in just a few short weeks. These routines will lead you down a path of healthy lifestyle transformation. The real gold is in how much better you will feel about yourself and your life as a whole.

Are you on board? Are you ready to become empowered? If so, go ahead and move on to chapter 2. If you aren't quite motivated to change your life yet, keep reading. Let's be frank: life is too short, and you don't have time to waste. You need to know the stakes of the game you are playing with yourself. Think about how your self-destructive behavior affects the people in your life who love and care about you. Stop for a moment and think about how your participation in any unhealthy, self-destructive behavior affects your loved ones, whether it be overeating, undereating, smoking, doing drugs, or abusing alcohol. If you are honest with yourself, you will realize that self-destructive behavior affects more than your health; it affects your relationships with others as well.

Self-sabotage is not limited to affecting your health. There is also a direct correlation with how much others respect you and want to be around you. Self-destructive behavior carries over into other areas of your life. Could you be sabotaging your close personal and business relationships? Could this kind of pattern appear in your work? Could similar behavior carry over into the way you care for yourself? Undoubtedly!

Let's talk facts for a minute. According to the surgeon general and the Centers for Disease Control and Prevention, the biggest threat to our health is no longer tobacco and smoking-related diseases. The biggest threat is inactivity and being overweight. Heart disease, diabetes, stroke, and many forms of cancer are directly linked to inactivity and obesity. Here are the numbers: more than 3 million Americans will die this year from diseases that could be prevented by regular exercise and sensible eating.

That is, on average, about 8,300 people each and every day. One of those people could be your mother or father, your sister or brother, your closest friend, your spouse, your child. It could be *you.*

Are you overweight and out of shape? Are you overwhelmed and stressed out? Are you often lethargic and exhausted? Do you frequently feel anxious or agitated? Are you not exercising or eating properly? If you said "yes" to any of these questions, please realize that your lifestyle supports it. You have chosen this for yourself. Don't you think it's time to start making better choices? Changing just one behavior has profound effects. Removing just one element of self-sabotage can create a domino effect of positive changes. Take this first step, and every aspect of your life can improve.

Let me be honest with you: the most difficult step in transforming your body and your life is making the choice to do so. You can choose not to be self-sabotaging, and you can choose a pattern of behavior that is not self-destructive. The choice is yours to make, but if you make the right choice the Body Express Makeover will support you all the way to the finish line.

It all comes down to fostering a deeper respect for yourself and learning to make caring for yourself a top priority. It is within your means. *You can do this!* But only you can choose to be healthy or not. You have to want it. Why wouldn't you? You can ponder the question for years, or you can have the courage to change your life now. The Body Express Makeover is *the* solution for the changes you want to make! I don't know if you have noticed yet, but I tend to be pretty direct and to the point. I don't believe in beating around the bush; I believe in tackling issues and problems that deter us head-on.

If any of us honestly looks in the rearview mirror of life, there is no great mystery of how or when we began putting on those extra pounds. It didn't happen overnight. It was either an issue that plagued us from childhood, or it happened slowly, over time. It is so common, so pervasive, that the scientific community has dubbed this problem "creeping obesity." The phenomenon of creeping obesity can be defined simply as a slow weight gain over several years. So if you have gained a pound or two a year since you graduated from high school or college, chances are that this extra weight represents the exact amount of weight you would now like to lose. The reason you gained those pounds is not a mystery. You didn't gain weight because of a decline in your "metabolism"; rather, you gained it because of a decrease in activity.

It's all about time . . . your decreased activity level is directly related to your increased level of responsibility. You simply haven't had the time for enough physical activity. As a recent graduate, you may have gotten your first job, and with that responsibility, you spent less time being active. As you advanced in the workplace, you began further limiting your activity time. Or as serious relationships, marriage, or children came into your life, your time for being active also decreased. The Body Express training system obliterates the excuse of not having enough time. You can get a complete total body workout in just ten minutes.

There are many people who become motivated to change only after some health-related event or crisis occurs. But you don't need to wait for a wake-up call from your body. Do it now. Don't wait for your body to start quitting on you. Unfortunately, most people choose to drastically alter their lifestyle only after the threat becomes crystal clear. They have lost control of their bodies and have come to realize the enormity of what they may be taking for granted. If you wait for your body to send you the signal, if you wait for your body's wake-up call, it just may be too late.

The U.S. Department of Health and Human Services oversees virtually every federally-funded health-related program in this country. Because the government provides funding for almost every health-related company, organization, hospital, university, and institution, this department distributes virtually all health-related information to our nation. Recently, Tommy Thompson, the former secretary of health and human services, provided us with the following important information:

> Regular physical activity, fitness, and exercise are critically important for the health and well-being of people of all ages. Research has demonstrated that virtually all individuals can benefit from regular physical activity, whether they participate in vigorous exercise or some type of moderate health-enhancing physical activity. Even among frail and old adults, mobility and functioning can be improved through physical activity. Therefore physical fitness should be a priority for all Americans.

Regular physical activity has been shown to reduce the mortality rate from many chronic diseases. Millions of Americans suffer from chronic illnesses and diseases that can be prevented or improved through regular physical activity:

- 12.6 million people have coronary heart disease.
- 1.1 million people suffer from a heart attack in any given year.
- 17 million people have diabetes; about 90 to 95 percent of cases are type 2 diabetes, which is associated with obesity and physical inactivity; approximately 16 million people have prediabetes.
- 107,000 people are diagnosed with colon cancer every year.
- 300,000 people suffer from hip fractures every year.
- 50 million people have high blood pressure.
- Nearly 50 million adults between the ages of 20 and 74, or 30 percent of the adult population, are obese; overall, more than 108 million adults, or 64.5 percent of the adult population, are overweight or obese.

In a 1993 study, 14 percent of all deaths in the United States were attributable to activity patterns and diet. Another study linked sedentary lifestyles to 23 percent of deaths from major chronic diseases. For example, physical activity has been shown to reduce the risk of developing or dying from heart disease, diabetes, colon cancer, and high blood pressure. On average, people who are physically active outlive those who are inactive.

> Participation in regular physical activity—at least thirty minutes of moderate activity at least five days per week, or twenty minutes of vigorous physical activity at least three

times per week—is critical to sustaining good health. You should strive for one hour of exercise every day. Regular physical activity has beneficial effects on most (if not all) organ systems, and consequently it helps prevent a broad range of health problems and diseases.

—Tommy Thompson

Regular physical activity reduces the risk of developing or dying from the leading causes of illness in the United States. Regular physical activity improves health in the following ways:

- It reduces the risk of dying prematurely from heart disease and other conditions.
- It reduces the risk of developing diabetes.
- It reduces the risk of developing high blood pressure.
- It reduces blood pressure in people who already have high blood pressure.
- It reduces the risk of developing colon and breast cancer.
- It helps maintain healthy weight.
- It helps build and maintain healthy bones, muscles, and joints.
- It helps older adults become stronger and better able to move without falling.
- It reduces feelings of depression and anxiety; and
- It promotes psychological well-being.

Again, I am very direct with my clients, and I will be very direct with you. Occasionally, I have my clients do tasks that I know will raise their motivation level a couple of notches. For example, I have one task that I give certain clients, and it works every time. I ask them to write a letter to someone they love. In that letter,

I ask them to explain to that person why they are no longer alive. I ask them to explain why they couldn't find ten or twenty minutes a day to get off their butts and exercise. I urge them to explain why they couldn't eat healthfully and take care of themselves. I then ask them to read it every time they don't want to work out. Does it work? Why don't you try it?

To whom will you write your letter? Your spouse, your child, your parents? Write that person a letter. Really, do it. Tell them all the reasons why you couldn't do this for yourself. Most likely what you will discover is a series of excuses a mile long that you actually had a choice in changing. Keep the letter in a place where you can access it easily, and read it every time you want to use some excuse for why you can't, shouldn't, or would rather not exercise. Read it every time you want to procrastinate. Read it every time you feel as though you deserve not to do what you know you should do. If you are honest with yourself, it should motivate you to choose life every time.

You have every chance to live a long, healthy life. With each passing decade, medical advances increase our chances of living longer lives. Today there are more people living beyond one hundred than at any other time in history, and according to recent studies this population segment is expected to increase by 40 percent in the next fifty years.

Take a look at an older person who is healthy, energetic, vital, and engaged in life. Does he or she have a zest for living? What is his or her mental state like? Is that person "positive"? Is he or she joyous? Is he or she still sharp and on top of things? Can he or she still care for him- or herself and find the time to care for others? Is that person someone you look up to and wish to emulate? If your answers were "yes," chances are that person is very active. He or she probably finds time to do some form of physical activity, whether it be walking, gardening or yard work, golf, tennis, or some other leisure activity that keeps him or her moving. Look at that person closely, and you will discover that his or her secret fountain of youth is most likely daily exercise or physical activity.

Exercise is the reason vibrant older people are positive and mentally sharp. It is very likely why they are joyous, engaged, and happy. If their peers are still living (ponder that for a moment), what is their quality of life? If they were no longer active, I would wager that their quality of life would be the polar opposite. Which person would you rather be? Sixty is young today. Sixty means you could have twenty to forty more incredible years! Finding some time for activity and taking care of yourself can add years to your life. Quality of life is really the whole point. Let's not waste any more time. Move past whatever contemplations you are having. Let go of all the false rationalizations for why you can't succeed in having the body you've always dreamed of having. Now is the time to take action, to get empowered, and to get on board the Body Express Makeover. I will tell you everything you need to do. Just do it! Throw yourself into the deep end. I promise you that you will swim. You will arrive at your ultimate destination. You will also find plenty of support at www.bodyexpressmakeover.com.

RAPID RESULTS

The Body Express is the fastest vehicle to take you where you need to go. The program will change your body rapidly and help you gain the confidence needed to support a healthy lifestyle transformation. My promise to you is that if you make the commitment and stay consistent, you will see

amazing results and be on the path to empowerment and success. I have seen it work with hundreds of my clients. This training system is simply the fastest, most effective way to get the body you want.

Like an actor, you want to see results in the way your body looks yesterday. Normally, actors are hired to portray a role and come in with the script. They will typically have anywhere from two weeks to three months before filming starts. More often than not, they will need to look dramatically different when shooting begins. During this short period of time, I work with them very closely. I create a nutrition strategy for them. I design a specific training regimen, and I spend many hours with them in the gym. Because I am by their side coaching them daily and can steer them through obstacles, their results are very dramatic.

The one quality that I would like you to emulate is their level of commitment. Celebrities are highly motivated, often because they are being paid a lot of money to look their best. Their intense motivation enables them to

achieve truly astounding results. But this degree of body transformation does not have to be limited to the rich and famous. Perhaps you have seen some of the less famous people I have worked with on the television show *Extreme Makeover*. These contestants underwent the most awe-inspiring process of transformation—on national television! They spent an average of two weeks working with me after having numerous cosmetic surgery procedures, but in that short amount of time they achieved monumental results and continue to build on the foundation we created together.

Anyone can do this! You can do it more quickly than you ever imagined! In fact, the quickest and most dramatic transformations I have overseen were accomplished by the people who had the farthest distance to travel. For them, the key was fortitude. Because they were diligent in chipping away at their personal mountain, not only did they achieve a new body, but they developed tools and skills that helped them create a new, more vital life.

EXTREME MAKEOVER TESTIMONIALS

DESHANTE

I feel that the time I spent with you for *Extreme Makeover* contributed a great deal to my transformation. I could not have done it without you. I thank you so much for your hard work and for working me hard! I am very grateful. Everyone else didn't get to see how much your efforts changed me. I thank God for my time with you. And I want you to know that you're amazing.

TAMMY

My reveal on *Extreme Makeover* went great! Everyone said that they wouldn't have even recognized me, so I guess that is good! I can't thank you enough for pushing me to work hard at the gym. You have helped bring a workout program back into my schedule. I rejoined the gym and have been getting my cardiovascular and weight training in almost every day. I feel great.

ANGELA

Michael was part of my *Extreme Makeover* dream team. His system of exercise and eating right absolutely works! I watched myself lose twenty pounds in just under four weeks, going from a size 14 to a size 8. Michael, you've helped my life physically and mentally. Thank you so much!!

Your Own Personal Coach

All of my celebrity clients and many contestants you may have seen on *Extreme Makeover* had one thing in common: me. If you were a client of mine, I would spend many hours with you in the gym every week, and then you would have homework to do on top of that. If you were on *Extreme Makeover*, I would be your personal coach, motivating and educating you. If I were by your side morning, noon, and night, I could do all of your planning and all of your programming, provide your motivation, and give you all the components you would need to reach your fitness goals fast. For every step you took to reach those goals, I would give you positive reinforcement and point out the results that had been achieved by taking each and every step.

However, we all know that I can't be there for you every step of the way. But the truth is that you can do the same thing just as efficiently and effectively on your own with the programs and guidance I provide in this book. You do not need a drill instructor; you simply need a little guidance to get you moving in the right direction. For the remainder of this chapter, I would like to teach you to become your own coach. More specifically, I would like to teach you how to coach yourself toward your health and wellness goals and to acknowledge the results you achieve along the way.

An important part of being your own coach is being able to separate truth from fallacy in the weight loss world. How are you supposed to reward yourself or evaluate your progress if you are unsure of what the facts are? There is an important fallacy that I would like to address because I know it plagues many of you. Whether this is the first time you've tried to transform your lifestyle or your twentieth, you have undoubtedly heard that in order to lose weight, you need willpower and self-discipline. I know it's not that simple. It's not so much having willpower and self-discipline as it is about your state of mind. Are you ready to do this? Are you truly ready to commit to this transformation? You can't control the physical cravings or triggers that will arise on occasion. None of us can!

But you *can* control how you will react to certain situations and mental states of mind. The mental aspect of losing weight is all about being in a state of mind that will not allow you to deviate from your ultimate goal—for any reason. In other words, your mental state of mind needs to be that not losing weight or reaching your ultimate goal is *not an option!* Having a state of mind that makes a stand and says that not achieving all your goals is *not an option* is overwhelmingly more powerful than relying on the uncontrollable—and much weaker—willpower or self-discipline alone.

I'm not saying you will not have setbacks along the way. You will. Let me repeat: you will have setbacks along the way. However, your success will rest on how well you react to them. In the past, you may have reacted to eating a meal that you knew was an unhealthy choice by finishing the rest of the day with bad food choices. That's usually the beginning of a downward spiral. Ultimately, it can lead to failure. But let's put it into perspective. If you eat an unhealthy meal, it was just that: one unhealthy meal. It doesn't turn into an unhealthy *day* of meals unless you *choose* to make it so. But if making that choice is *not an option,* you just acknowledge having that meal, note it, and move on. You see how having a state of mind that says "No" to failure keeps you accountable to yourself? I don't want you to beat yourself up every time you have a setback. On the flip side, I don't want you to let yourself off the hook either. Just acknowledge any mistakes you may make and move on. Don't give them any power they shouldn't have or, more important, power over your mental state of mind.

How many times have you had a bad morning and somehow your whole day ended up as a "bad day"? I can almost guarantee that you left your house in a mental state of mind that left you open to having that "bad day." The truth is, you can spill coffee on your freshly pressed shirt while you're running late and still have a good day. An unhealthy lunch doesn't mean an unhealthy eating day; it just means you had an unhealthy lunch. A missed workout doesn't mean a bad workout week; it just means you missed a workout. It's important to keep things in perspective and not blow them out of proportion. A very wise friend once told me, "Michael, having a bad day does not mean you have a bad life, it just means you had a bad day." Ignite your own internal power by choosing a mental state that will not allow you to get derailed; it's *not an option.*

Tools of Transformation

Becoming your own best coach will require some basic tools. There are two simple tools that I suggest using to *track your results* and *achieve your goal:* a calendar and a journal of some kind. Your journal can be any shape or size but should be a fixture on your bed stand or night table. Your calendar should optimally be a bound book that displays each week over two pages.

While these tools have a simple function, what is written in them will reflect your thoughts, feelings, and experiences during your journey. Your journal has a dual purpose. It will be the place where you write down your goals, hopes, dreams, feelings, and tangible visualizations that encompass all your fitness goals. It will also act as the receptacle of your results, and you will use it often to make brief notes on how you progress and how you feel after your workouts. Utilizing a journal will hold you accountable to yourself, just as I hold my clients accountable to me. Because so many of your results will be realized within—increased self-confidence and mental clarity, more energy throughout the day, sleeping better at night—where no one else can see the change, it is essential that you catalog your results for your own personal review. The calendar will act as your personal planner and enable you to become the master of your greatest resource: your time. It will also become the road map you use to trace each step on the road to your ultimate destination.

Journal

You have already taken the first step and conquered the first stage of change, which is pre-contemplation. You have decided to embark upon a journey to change your body. You are already midstride in the second step of changing your body and your life, which is the process of contemplation. The best tool for this contemplation is your journal. I always suggest using this journal for at least six weeks, but I encourage you to use it for as long as you feel the need.

I want you to start by dividing your journal into four separate sections. The first section will be titled "Notes to Self." This is where you will write down your ultimate goal, your immediate goals, your strategies to achieve them, and your visualizations. No, this is not some New Age, metaphysical book; however, I will have you do some visualization exercises because they are extremely powerful tools of change. How can you have the body of your dreams unless you can vi-

sualize what it will look like? When you get dressed for work in the morning and you are choosing your wardrobe, don't you visualize, sometimes unconsciously, what you would look like in a certain outfit before you put it on and step in front of the mirror? You will also write down your feelings and thoughts after each workout. How did you feel immediately after exercising? Writing down your feelings and observations will help you stay the course and motivate you on days when you don't feel like exercising.

The second section will be titled "Aerobic Training." This is where you will write down what form of cardiovascular activity you did and how long you did it each and every time you do it.

The third section will be titled "2-in-1 Training." This is where you will write down which 2-in-1 Strength Training routine you did (the 10, 20, or 30).

The last section will be titled "Nutrition." At the end of each day, you will write down how well you adhered to your nutrition strategy. You can use this section in a way that works best for you from a time and creative standpoint. You don't necessarily have to write down each and every food item you eat. I will leave it up to you to do what works best for you personally.

The purpose of keeping this journal is twofold. First, it will be used to keep you accountable to yourself. And second, it will be necessary later in the book when we get to the reward system that you will be following. Yes, there are ways to make exercising a little more fun and interesting, and a reward system is the perfect way to do so.

Believe it or not, just by getting past the

first chapter and making the commitment to change your body, you have already begun the process of healthy lifestyle transformation and overcome the first stage of change: precontemplation. But where should you go from here? We will begin with baby steps. These small steps will lead to strides, and these strides will lead to leaps and bounds. The next step is important and includes purchasing another journal. You can use an inexpensive spiral-bound notebook or an expensive leather-bound one; it does not matter. If you don't have one, please get one before you read any further. It is an important part of the program that can't be overlooked.

I would like you always to have this journal on or near you during the day, so that you can make notations of anything that strikes you. I would also encourage you to get into the habit of setting it on your bedside table each night. You need some alone time for this exercise, so if you share your bedroom, find a quiet place without disruptions or distractions. When you are settled in, I would like you to close your eyes and really try to visualize how you would like your body to look. I want you to picture yourself getting undressed, looking in the mirror, and seeing your body transformed. I want you to stay with this image until it becomes palpable, until you can really sense what it would be like to have it. Take your time.

When this image of your new self becomes ingrained in your mind, I would like you to turn to the first page of your journal under the "Notes to Self" section and write down some impressions of the vision you just had. You don't have to be a novelist or poet, just provide some detail of what you just saw in your mind's eye.

Start with the big picture: How did you look overall? (Instead of writing "I was" please write, "I am.") What features or body parts were most notable? When you saw yourself in the mirror, what was different about your personality? Did the person in the mirror act differently? Did you carry yourself differently or seem to have any personality traits that are different from your present ones? Write down other nontangible qualities you visualized, such as less stressed, well rested, or increased energy levels. Answer these simple questions and expand upon them if you wish, but do not edit your thoughts.

So that was it. That was your second step. You have just contemplated what you would like to achieve. Just doing this exercise will tell you a great deal about what your goals really are. This exercise will also tell you how well you take direction, how motivated you are, the level of your desire to change, and your capacity for self-discipline. But what it will also tell you is how prominent your negative self-talk is. If you chose not to purchase a journal for yourself and/or did not do the visualization exercise, it's not too late. Really, *do the exercise*—this is a significant step.

Once you complete the visualization exercise, you are well on your way to achieving your dream body. If you haven't written down your vision, you need to ask yourself why you are unwilling to do an activity that will provide the foundation of your success. When we write down our vision, goals, and thoughts, we are literally making a commitment to ourselves to follow through with our intentions. If you were traveling in a foreign country, wouldn't you buy a road map to guide you? Well, your journal provides a similar function in that it is a motivational support tool that you will refer back to when you need to be reminded of your goal. Your journal will reaffirm your vision and empower you to remain committed despite obstacles. Not having a journal would be like attempting to put together a complicated home entertainment center without the instructions. Everyone needs support and a process that has a proven track record. So take a moment to do the visualization exercise and record your thoughts in your journal. If you have already followed the directions, found a quiet place, done the exercise, and written down the answers, congratulations! You will be seeing that new image in the mirror in the very near future.

Each and every day, you will strive to look and feel more like the *you* in your vision. Every night before you go to sleep, I would like you to repeat this exercise. It should be the last journal entry of the day. What you are striving to accomplish is to actualize, to make real, to personify, and to own this self-image. The more this vision becomes real to you, the more you will own it. Owning your vision is saying "Yes" to changing your body and your lifestyle.

The more consistent you are with your journal, the more valuable the exercise will become. Why is that? Because it's consistency in exercise and healthful eating that encourages the formation of a daily habit and promotes long-term success. If you can stick to using your journal daily, you will be much more likely to adhere to consistent exercise and healthful eating. I encourage you to make brief notations after every workout. If there is a time in your day when you usually experience a drop-off in energy or an "afternoon slump," I suggest you take a five-minute break and make a note about it in your journal. Some days you might see a change in the way a particular body part looks or notice your clothes becoming looser in the thighs, buttocks, or waist. On other days, these changes could be experiential—things that are not seen, but felt. These feelings and experiences are very real indeed, and because they are less tangible than your pants or dress size, it is essential that you write them down in your journal. As you become more aware of the experiential changes you are feeling, you will soon discover that you are becoming more like the *you* in your vision.

Calendar

You have seen the end result, the *ultimate goal,* the ideal you are striving for, and now you must do some planning to get there. In short, you must look at your *ultimate goal,* the image of yourself you saw in your mind's eye, and work backward to determine what it will take to reach that destination.

I have done much of the work for you, and I will guide you toward that plan. I will give you all the information you need to determine the "how" and "why," but you are responsible for the "when." I will coach you on exactly what you need to do and give you choices so you can personalize the program for yourself. However, it is your responsibility actually to carve out some time in your daily schedule. I have done everything in my power to make your workouts the ultimate in time efficiency, but realizing your vision of yourself requires planning so that you can fit it into your day.

As I've said before, time is the number one

obstacle in the way of your attaining your vision. Your journal will provide the black-and-white controls of how stringent and consistent you are on your new path. However, to eliminate the obstacle of time, you will need to plan ahead. This is exactly what I tell my clients day in and day out: *Plan ahead.* This is where many people sabotage their weight loss and healthy lifestyle efforts. By not planning ahead, you end up in situations where you are forced to eat poorly or not exercise due to time constraints. Don't fall into this trap. This is the fastest way to spiral downward because not having time can be rationalized as a realistic excuse every time unless you plan ahead. If time is your number one obstacle, then planning ahead is your number one solution.

I'm not saying that life won't throw you curve balls. We both know it will. But planning will dramatically reduce the number of times you have slips. When you decide to go on a vacation, do you plan the trip, or do you just hop into your car or board a plane without a destination? That's exactly my point. A successful, relaxing, joyful vacation has to be planned, and so should a new exercise program.

To plan ahead, you will need some sort of calendar. It can be an electronic version, a wall calendar, or a desktop month-by-month calendar. It is important to use it every day. Not only will it help you plan when you will eat, exercise, and run errands such as grocery shopping, it will also help you with time management in other areas of your life and show you where you might be squandering time that could be better utilized. Trust me, I understand busy schedules. My schedule can be nonstop from 7 A.M. to 8 P.M., but I use a daily, weekly, and monthly calendar to plan everything, including my workouts. I rarely miss a workout or a meal. This tool allows me to have structure. Structure provides balance in life that reduces and eliminates stress and self-sabotage.

Every Sunday night, I sit down with my planner and plan everything for the upcoming week. I plan my meetings, appointments, and every strength training and aerobic workout. I also plan when I am going to go grocery shopping and when I will do my food preparation for the upcoming week. I lay it all out for myself. I suggest that you do the same thing. Structure is the key to achieving the body you envision.

I want you to set aside one day during your weekend. I suggest Sunday. I want you to take that day as a leisure day, a day of recuperation, a day of fun activity. On that day, you should give yourself a part of the day to be outdoors. Go to the park or the beach, take a scenic walk, hike, ski, skate, ride your bike, play tennis or catch, go kayaking, or garden; it really doesn't matter what. Just make the activity something that you look forward to and that takes you away from your normal weekday routine. I find that spending a few hours at the beach or hiking in the mountains can feel like a minivacation. It helps me regroup, reflect, clear my head. It allows me to focus on what I need to do in the upcoming week.

Don't get me wrong, your life won't always go as planned. Life happens. But what this weekly exercise will do is provide you with a structure. This structure will not only enable you to be more effective, but it will allow you to become more flexible when things do not go according to plan. This structure will reinforce the new priority in your life and provide a format to make time for it.

Rapid Results

You want results. Over the years I have been asked hundreds of times, "How do you stay motivated to exercise consistently?" The answer is always the same: *Results! Results! Results!* When you see and feel changes in your body and consistently have positive feelings about yourself, you will be motivated to continue realizing those very results. You want results. You want immediate gratification. You want to look a certain way, and you want to look that way now. Great. That is fantastic motivation to get you started. Hang on to it. However, if you don't look the way you want to in a week or two, you may get disappointed. You need to discover something even greater to keep you coming back and pushing forward. You will never, ever look the way you want to look if you quit. In this process, the benefits you gain every day add up exponentially and will be more valuable than the riches you receive by getting to that final destination. So I urge you to be very clear about what *goals* you would like to achieve, and what kind of *results* you want to experience.

Goals Versus Results

Let's get clear about your goals. You want the perfect body and you want it now . . . but let's be realistic. If you have fifty pounds to lose, it's going to take some time. I know you've heard this before, but there are no quick fixes. If you think that is disappointing, I have good news and great news. The good news is that you can

and will get the body you want. The great news is that because it will take time to get the body of your dreams, you will attain something even greater during that period.

I would wager that getting a new body is only part of what you really want. I would wager that there is much, much more to your ultimate goal. I'll be more specific. You envisioned yourself with the body of your dreams; what would it mean to have the body of your dreams? Get past the vanity issues; looks are truly skin deep. That may sound strange coming from a trainer. But this book is about more than that. The *you* in your vision feels different than you do now. That *you* carries him- or herself differently and with more confidence. What else would you gain by achieving your goal? It could be a whole host of things that we associate with "quality of life": overall improved health, more energy, better sleep, a positive outlook on life, stronger bones, stronger heart, improved stamina, better sex, greater respect, or more power. If you are being honest with yourself, you undoubtedly want more than washboard abs and a tight tush. *You want a better life.*

There is a vast difference between results and goals, and it is important that you make the distinction between the two. The Body Express Makeover is about a process, a journey to reach that destination—your ultimate *goal.* What will happen along that journey is just as important as reaching the destination. What will happen along the path of your personal journey is the experiential feelings of becoming that new person—the *you* you are striving to become. The experiential feelings that arise during this process and along this path are the *results.* Remember, the important thing is not having a perfect body, it's about feeling good in the body you have and being realistic about what you can achieve.

Goals

Let's stay with the *you* in your vision. I don't want to minimize what it means to attain your dream body. Getting that body means improving your life. However, the process of getting there is just as important. For the moment, let's imagine that the body you saw in your vision is your *goal*. That is your ultimate destination. It is the direction in which you are headed and for which you are striving. Now let's take that vision a step further.

I want you to see past your vision. I would like your ultimate goal to be getting your body to a place of maintenance. In other words, maintaining the body of your dreams for the rest of your life should be your goal. Your ultimate goal, then, is to reach the termination stage of change. Attaining this goal is a process that requires time; however, you will feel better and experience significant results along the way. These results will help you stick to your plan of action until you reach your destination. They are the reinforcing milestones that will continually motivate you to reach your goal.

Setting Realistic and Attainable Goals

Reason is the key to creating a goal that is based on realistic expectations. Part of our ability to reason means we need to deal with reality. There are many myths that need to be dispelled so that you have realistic expectations of what you can

and will achieve versus unrealistic expectations that will always be self-defeating.

There is an old saying, "It is better to shoot for the moon and reach the stars than to shoot for the stars and land on your butt." The exact opposite is true here. You do yourself no good at all when you set unattainable goals. The great thing about goals is that once they are achieved, you can always create new ones. As an example, let's say you have 100 pounds to lose. Wanting to lose 100 pounds is fine; however, doesn't that sound much more daunting than, say, losing 20 pounds? Losing 100 pounds is a huge goal and could be too far away to be able to visualize realistically. However, if you make losing 20 pounds your immediate goal and strive to lose 1 to 2 pounds per week, you could realistically achieve this goal, and it would be less daunting because you can actually visualize it. Once achieved, the next 20 pounds might be even less daunting, and that would give way to eventually losing the last 60 pounds. You would be less likely to be derailed, and soon you would be 100 pounds lighter. Maybe you'll find that you are happy losing only 50 pounds or that losing only 60 pounds is realistic for your body type and lifestyle. As you achieve each of these smaller, more realistic goals, your confidence will increase and your chances of being successful will be far greater.

The key here is to take baby steps. Many times we unconsciously sabotage ourselves by taking on a goal that is too big. When we fail, it once again proves that we cannot lose weight or sculpt our body. Then we punish ourselves for not being able to achieve our weight loss goals, and many times we gain even more weight. Be kind to yourself and make your time frame for attaining your fitness goals realistic. Henry Ford didn't become the largest auto manufacturer in a day; he started by making one car at a time.

In line with being realistic, there are genetic limitations that you may not be able to overcome. It is just a reality that you might never be a size 2. If you have a 42-inch waistline, it may be physically impossible to have a 28-inch waist. Clients have come to me and said, "I want to lose ten pounds" when they don't have 10 pounds of body fat to lose. You need to be realistic about what you can attain with your body structure and lifestyle. Of course, there are exceptions to every rule, but the point is to be realistic and honest with yourself.

Many of us are searching for a "magic bullet," a miracle cure that will give us the body we want. That is a fairy tale. It doesn't exist. It never has, and it never will. Part of being realistic means that you have to shut out the hype that we are bombarded with every day. More than 60 percent of the people in this country are overweight or obese, and weight loss is a multibillion-dollar industry. If you are overweight, advertisers have painted a target on your forehead and will do anything to get you to buy their product. Many of the products you see advertised in periodicals, tabloid newspapers, and e-mails use very deceptive practices. Because the FDA does not regulate nutritional supplements, diet pills, creams, potions, and powders can contain nearly anything. The great majority of these products do not work.

When enough people get together and bring a class-action suit against a company that sells such products, it happily pays a $5 million fine to the FCC for false advertising, declares bankruptcy, and transfers the $100 million it

made on the product into its bank account in the Cayman Islands. Then it takes some of that money, creates a new company, puts out another "new" product that probably doesn't work, and does the whole thing over again. Another practice many companies participate in is the usage of those *amazing* "before-and-after" photographs. Many of the "perfect" bodies that you see in magazines are airbrushed. If you are looking at an advertisement for a weight loss product, many times the photos have been retouched or doctored in some way. How do we know how long it took the person in the photo to look that way, and what proof do we have that he or she actually used that product to get that physique in the first place?

Being realistic about your dream body means getting rid of the notion that you need to have a "perfect body." There simply is no such thing. I have worked with some of the most beautiful people in Hollywood, whose bodies are admired by millions, and believe me, none of them is completely satisfied with the way he or she looks. Just like you, they would all like to change something about their appearance. You can never achieve the perfect body. Trying to do so becomes an obsessive and quite insane quest for the unattainable. What you can achieve, what your goal should be, is to create a body that makes you feel good and that ultimately fits into your lifestyle. It should be realistic based upon your genetic profile, age, and fitness condition.

The Lies Your Scale Tells

When you are determining your fitness goals, I want you to be very careful about projecting a desired weight. The biggest myth about changing your body can be dispelled when you throw away your scale. Your progress should not be measured on the scale. The scale is not a fair indicator of your progress, and it should not have anything to do with reaching your goal.

The scale cannot and will not tell you what you want to know. For instance, if you have been sedentary and have not exercised for many years (if ever), and you begin exercising regularly, your overall weight might not go down for some time. Because muscle weighs twice as much as fat, your weight might actually increase for a few weeks; but since you are adding lean muscle mass, you are getting stronger and raising your metabolic rate so that you are burning calories (fat) more efficiently. After the next few weeks, your weight on the scale might begin to drop again, but that is still a false indicator of your progress. Your weight can fluctuate up to 3 pounds daily based upon the last time you ate, your salt intake, your water retention, and your last elimination. I'm not saying your overall weight is not important. What I'm saying is to stop obsessing about it. The weight—or, better yet, body fat—will come off in time. Using a scale can be very deceiving and discouraging if done obsessively.

On the Body Express training system, you will be adding lean muscle mass. When you reach your ultimate goal or maintenance phase, you might actually weigh as much on the scale as you do now, but you will be wearing clothes that are several sizes smaller. To get past what the scale says, I suggest you think about this: If you weighed 10 pounds more than you do right now but were four sizes smaller, would you really care how much you weighed? No! In short, your weight on the scale is only a small part of the big picture. Trust that your weight will drop along with your body fat percentage if you follow the Body Express Makeover system.

How Do I Measure My Results?

The best method to chart your progress is by determining your body fat percentage. This process can be simple or complicated, cheap or very expensive. It can be done with a $5 caliper by taking various measurements from different body parts, or it can be done by a method called bioimpedance, where you stand on or hold a device that sends an electric charge through your body. It can be done by immersion or by the very expensive high-tech methods used by NASA on astronauts. Some methods are more accurate than others. Many gyms and alternative medical facilities have a person on staff who can do this measurement for you for about $15. The most important thing is to use the same method at the same time of day, under the same conditions.

This is how body fat measurement works, and this is what it will tell you. First, you will weigh yourself on the scale (one of the only times I promote getting on a scale). What you really want to know and determine is: How much of that weight is made up of lean muscle, and how much of that weight is made up of bones, hair, and water? Last, how much of that weight is made up of fat? The trick is to lose body fat, not muscle.

If you added one pound of muscle and did not lose any fat, you would be a pound heavier on the scale, *but* you would automatically have a lower percentage of body fat. Do you want less bone density? No! You want your bones to increase in density. As we age, we become susceptible to osteoporosis, a severe reduction of bone density and structural deterioration of bone tissue. Our bones become less dense and have a tendency to break more easily. In the U.S., 10 million people already have some stage of osteoporosis. One in two women and one in four men over the age of fifty will experience an osteoporosis fracture. Exercise that utilizes resistance or weight training will increase the density of your bones, and the training system outlined in this book will expedite the process.

How Often Should I Measure Myself?

There are two rules of thumb when it comes to taking measurements. I'm not a big proponent of taking measurements often. If you are within 15 pounds of your ideal weight, your clothes are really the best indicator of what's happening with your body. However, if you are 30 pounds or more overweight, taking measurements periodically, say every four to six weeks, can motivate you to stay on track. Also, if you tend to be a very visual person and feel a need to measure periodically, go ahead and do so. However, you should not measure more than every four to six weeks because the body needs time to register a change that is dramatic enough to be motivational. Every time you measure, you would like to see your percentage of lean muscle *increase* and the percentage of your total weight made up of body fat *decrease.* Please understand that it may take several weeks before your metabolism kicks into high gear, so don't get discouraged if you don't see external changes fast enough. In-

ternal changes are taking place. I promise it will happen.

How Much Fat Can I Lose, and How Fast Can I Lose It?

There are many factors that contribute to the question "How fast?" Your diet, how long you have been sedentary, and whether or not you have been physically active at some point in your life are all very definitive variables in the time factor of this process. In some ways, the speed and pace at which you lose weight is very much like riding a bike. Your body has some level of cellular and muscle memory and after being reoriented can get back into the swing of things, just as you can when getting on a bicycle after several years of not riding. At first you might be a little unsteady, but very soon your body will remember what to do. The same is true of your body and the transformation process.

If you have exercised previously, you will most likely realize increased muscle tone and shape faster than someone who has not. You will quickly see your level of endurance and overall fitness condition return to what you may have once enjoyed. If you have not exercised for a few years or at all, you may have to start out slowly, and it may take longer to see results. However, if you are consistent, over time your body will kick into high gear and you will see changes happen almost overnight. The keys here are *patience* and *consistency.* It is entirely possible that your results will go through peaks and valleys. You may see great results for a few weeks and then notice hardly anything for the next couple of weeks. Don't get discouraged. What is happening on the inside of your body takes time to be reflected on the outside. This is where trust in the process and your coach comes into play. It all depends on one thing: if you are diligent about eating healthfully and exercising consistently, you will see dramatic changes in your appearance very quickly.

Everyone has a certain percentage of body fat, which is essential to a myriad of bodily functions. Men such as professional athletes, marathon runners, and bodybuilders can get their body fat percentage down under 10 percent. The very fittest have between 3 percent and 7 percent body fat. If you can reduce your body fat to 20 percent—you will look and feel extraordinary. For women, these percentages are higher and, for many health reasons, should be. Female athletes may get their body fat percentage down to the 10 to 17 percent range but may experience health-related issues as a result. The loss or irregularity of their menstrual cycle, a reduction in bone density, and eating disorders are the three symptoms of a phenomenon called female triad syndrome. This syndrome plagues many female athletes and sets off a chain reaction of even greater health problems. In extreme cases, women in their twenties have the bone density of eighty-year-olds and are highly susceptible to breaking bones if they fall, jog, or jump. For them, childbirth (if it is even possible) can be a life-threatening event. It is far better that you set your sights on a body fat percentage of 20 percent.

Following is an example of a typical BMI chart. Keep in mind that the BMI chart is to be used only as a general guideline.

Realistically, you can lose 1 to 2 pounds of fat per week, the average being 1.5 pounds. If

BMI CHART		
Adults	Women	Men
anorexia	<17.5	
underweight	<19.1	<20.7
in normal range	19.1–25.8	20.7–26.4
marginally overweight	25.8–27.3	26.4–27.8
overweight	27.3–32.3	27.8–31.1
very overweight or obese	>32.3	>31.1
severely obese	35–40	
morbidly obese	40–50	
super obese	50–60	

you are really pushing, you may be able to lose more, but it's important to pace yourself or you may have difficulty sustaining such a high tempo and risk "burnout." I have seen this time and time again. How many of you are guilty of making the infamous New Year's resolution and then going from 0 to 100 in just a few short weeks? All of a sudden you begin feeling lethargic, you find it hard to wake up in the morning, and you get frustrated at not seeing your body change fast enough. You start asking yourself the proverbial question: Is this really worth all the effort I'm putting into it? These are all symptoms of burnout. If burnout causes you to stop dead in your tracks, you can easily gain back much of the weight you have lost. A very important key to remember is that consistency in weight loss is more important than speed. I implore you to pace yourself and cannot emphasize enough that if you can reduce 1 to 2 pounds of body fat per week, you are right on track. The body has its own time clock when it comes to weight reduction. You did not gain that extra 10, 20, or 30 pounds in a few weeks, so you can't expect it to come off in just a few weeks.

Can I Choose Where I Lose?

Spot reduction is a myth. You cannot eliminate fat from areas of your choosing. It doesn't work that way. The body responds as it wants to and you can't control that; but please keep in mind that while you cannot spot reduce, you can spot *tone* once your body fat is reduced.

Unfortunately, the first place you put on fat will generally be the last place it leaves. When you begin reducing your body fat percentage, there is no predicting where you will first notice that loss. Many of my female clients see a reduction in breast size. A client of mine made the cover of *Woman's World* magazine for going from a size 16 to a size 6 and losing 65 pounds in the process in approximately six months. However, she also lost four bra cup sizes. It wasn't exactly her first choice as to where to lose body fat, but she was also much happier and more positive. At first, your body fat reduction may be dramatic and may occur in odd places. But over time your weight loss will even out.

Taking baby steps is the key to achieving your dream, but again, this dream needs to be realistic. Remember your vision of yourself? It is important to check that vision against the reality of what you can actually achieve. You must first focus on a body that would make you feel comfortable and proud. Now open your journal to the "Notes to Self" section and take a look at some of the goals you wrote down earlier. Are they realistic and attainable? You may find that you need to make some adjustments. Go ahead and make those adjustments in your journal now if you need to.

Timeline

It's time to create a timeline to achieve your dream body and a healthy lifestyle. Once again, go to the "Notes to Self" section. How much body fat do you think you would need to lose to achieve the results you just wrote down? How long will it take you to reach this goal? Remember, at most, you should lose about 1 to 2 pounds of body fat per week. If you were aiming for 3 pounds per week, tone it down a bit and shoot for 2. If it has been a while since you were active, or if you have had difficulty adhering to a nutrition plan in the past, I want you to set the bar a little lower. If you were originally aiming for a loss of 2 pounds per week, shoot for 1. For example, let's pretend that your goal was to lose a total of 20 pounds of body fat; I would like you to achieve this objective in ten to twenty weeks (which is 1 to 2 pounds per week).

Okay, now open your calendar. When are you going to begin? Give yourself a few days to read the remainder of this book. **Put a star on your start date.** On that day, **pencil in a ten-minute block of time** for your first 2-in-1 strength workout. Now flip ahead and **draw another star on the date when you wish to reach your goal.**

Now you have a mission; you've set goals and an objective. Over the next few chapters, I will teach you how to plan, adhere to, and realize your goals and ultimately be successful.

Contract

Now open your journal and turn to the next blank page in the "Notes to Self" section. I want you to construct a commitment contract to yourself. You can devise this contract any way you desire, but here is a template to utilize if you can't come up with a contract that fits your needs:

I, _____ (name of reader), choose to live a healthy lifestyle. I choose to exercise consistently and to adhere to a healthful nutrition structure that will help me attain all of my health and wellness goals. I am committed to changing my lifestyle and to eating properly and exercising consistently. It is my goal to lose _____ pounds of body fat in _____ weeks. I will begin on _____ (date) and achieve my goal on _____ . I will do everything in my power to achieve this goal for myself. I owe it to myself. I will not quit until I achieve this goal. I will not let anything get in the way of my success. I will set realistic goals and hold myself accountable. This is my promise to myself. Not fullfilling my promise to myself is *not an option*!

(signature) _____

Look at these words in your journal. You have just made a commitment contract with yourself. I want you to make this contract binding. You can do that by sharing it with family and friends and asking for their support. Ask them for their support. Tell them that the best way they can support you is to not tempt you with foods or activities that could derail you. I also want you to make several copies of this contract and post them in places where you will be in daily contact with them. Post them in your bathroom, office, locker, address book; it

doesn't matter where you post them, just make sure this contract is in your face daily. You will need to be as passionate about reaching your fitness goals as I am in helping you reach them. I will provide you with all the information and tools you need to get there, but I want you to make it a top priority. From the day you start to the date you have set to reach your goals, I want this program to have the precedence it deserves. Do not let yourself down. Really go for it. Jump into the deep end, and do not let anything get in your way.

I promise that every step you take toward your ultimate goal will provide you with an infinite number of benefits, if you are willing to take notice. You will begin to feel better about yourself. You will be more energized. You will be more empowered. When you feel and see these results, I want you to write them down in your journal. These results are the very things that will keep you on track until you reach your ultimate goal.

Every day that you use the Body Express Makeover training system, you will be strengthening several personal characteristics. Your self-esteem and self-confidence will improve, giving you a more positive outlook on life. These are the things that give your life quality and are the inner tools of success. Over the next few chapters, I will remind you of these qualities and give you guidance on how to develop them, but for the moment, I just want to point them out to you so you can recognize them and begin the development of what I call "Power Tools."

These "Power Tools" are the tools you use in life to succeed and achieve. As you experience physical results, you will also experience inner growth. This is what is coming your way, and it's what I want you to be on the lookout for. You will experience a unification of *mind and body* and feel more whole. Ultimately, you will feel more grounded and together. You will experience a life-altering *shift*. This shift will affect your entire persona and positively impact every aspect of your life. Part of this shift will result in feeling as though you are *empowered*. You will begin to feel empowered emotionally, intellectually, and physically. This will result in an increase of *energy*, and you will *realize stress reduction* and *offset depression and negative self-talk*. Your level of *awareness* will dramatically increase. You will become more *centered* and more *present,* you will feel more *open,* and you will eventually become very turned on by the mindset of *possibility.* In the end, you will discover and strike a *balance* in your life. You will find peace and harmony within yourself. Isn't that really your ultimate goal? These feelings of well-being are just as important as having the body of your dreams.

The Mind/Body Connection

Whether you are conscious of it or not, you have already begun to synchronize your mind and body. By finishing the first chapter and reading on, you have made a commitment to yourself. In choosing to do what you know you should be doing, you have built a bridge between mind and body. This bridge will strengthen and expand as you progress. By making the conscious mental choice to change your body and your lifestyle, you have eliminated subconscious inner conflict. Your mind and body are now united to achieve a common objective. This is no small or trivial occurrence. This is a life-changing, life-affirming step, and you should acknowledge it. This one small decision has already changed your life and will continue to do so in a number of ways.

You are eliminating the saboteur from your life. Having decided to take positive action to improve your life, you have immediately become empowered, and you have said "yes" to life. Your conscious and subconscious are now in harmony. They are working together.

The great majority of your transformation will not happen through developing bigger biceps or tighter abs. Your transformation will become reality because of what happens between your ears. Your mind, your thoughts, your intentions, your will, and your intellect will have a great deal of power in this process. Every time you do your aerobic activities or perform your exercise routines, you will have the opportunity to strengthen the bridge between mind and body.

Shift

In choosing to eliminate the saboteur, by uniting mind and body to achieve a common goal, a dramatic inner shift is occurring. You might not feel this shift immediately, but each day you stay on course you may become more aware of it. In just a few short weeks or months, you will feel a sea change, a dynamic, dramatic paradigm shift throughout your entire persona.

This shift will not happen overnight; it is a process. It is very much like learning a new language. You begin by learning sentence structure, nouns and verbs and tenses. As you increase your vocabulary, you soon become able to put simple sentences together. As you begin to see progress, you are encouraged to practice more frequently. Before you know it, you become more and more fluent. The shift that is occurring in you now is similar to learning and using a new language. Eventually the new language becomes second nature. It is the same with exercising and healthful eating. They, too, will become second nature for you, just like brushing your teeth in the morning. You don't have to think about your commitment, you just do it. The more you utilize the Body Express Makeover training system, the greater your progress and the greater the shift will be. The greater the shift, the more positive changes you will realize in your life.

Activated

Physical activity is the key that will help unlock the doors to your personal growth and activate you on emotional, intellectual, and spiritual levels. Being physically active is the means by which you will achieve your goals.

When you get your body moving, miraculous things happen. When you exercise, a physiological change takes place. A natural hormonal release occurs, and the flood of hormones changes your chemical composition. Among these hormones are neuropeptides, adrenaline, and endorphins, which change you on a cellular level. When these hormones are released, you feel a sense of euphoria, which brings about a reduction of stress.

If you are facing personal adversity or have a negative outlook on life, you can reverse it.

When you are upset or experience high levels of stress, your body releases hormones that are damaging to your health and well-being on a cellular level. When a hormone such as cortisol, referred to as the stress hormone, is released in high enough quantities, it can cause a cellular disruption or disturbance. Interestingly, a high cortisol level also inhibits the loss of body fat. However, when you exercise, another flood of hormones is released that helps balance your hormonal levels. Striking this hormonal balance is the goal. As a result, you will be better equipped to handle stress and challenges. According to the Centers for Disease Control, conditions such as depression, the "blues," and negative thoughts and feelings can be drastically decreased, if not eliminated, by consistent exercise.

Energy

The combination of the beneficial release of hormones and the increase in circulation results in an increase of energy. You may feel exhausted prior to exercising but completely energized after a workout. Exercise is simply the best way to feel alert and rejuvenated. When we get upset, it drains us of energy. We feel tired, lethargic, and sleepy. Exercise can change that. The more you exercise, the more engaged you become. The more engaged you are in your life, the more energy you will have. This may be one of the biggest changes you will see over the course of your journey. No matter how much of a "couch potato" you may be, no matter how sedentary your lifestyle, you may just discover that there is a dynamo inside of you. With exercise, you can unleash that dynamo on the world.

Clarity

Another benefit you will experience will be clarity or a feeling of being clearheaded. You don't even have to wait until you finish exercising! Since stress is reduced by exercise, you will feel a little lighter in spirit. This lightening of spirit will give you a different perspective on your day and will, over time, begin to have this effect on your life as a whole. This change in perspective, this clearheadedness and clarity of thought, will enable you to make better decisions in your life. It will allow you to deal with life more effectively.

All of us have qualities about ourselves that we love. We all wish that those qualities were consistently in high gear. But the reality is that most of us are faced with issues at the most inopportune times. The same goes for me. Believe it or not, I make many of my most important decisions during my cardio sessions. If I need to make an important decision or am faced with some kind of personal crisis, I try not to worry, pace, or wring my hands. I put on my tennis shoes and go to the gym. After a few minutes of working out, my mind begins to slow down. Eventually, it slows down enough that I can see the bigger picture, making it easier to make decisions based on fact rather than emotion. Typically, by the end of my workout, I become closer to or have made a decision or realized that the situation is not as bad as I originally thought. I am ready to take whatever action is necessary to resolve the problem. My mind becomes so clear, so focused, that I am better equipped to see the situation for what it really is. When I don't have anything pressing me, I find that I am at my creative best because my mind is clear of clutter.

Centered

Being centered is a feeling of being grounded within yourself and in control of your emotions and your life. It suggests that you are rooted and anchored. Your personal "center" is the person you are when you are most content and balanced; it is your essence and deepest truth.

Any physical activity will effect a hormonal release and cause you to feel more centered. My programs utilize a training system made up of exercises that work your entire body in progression. The sequence of this progression and the complexity of some movements will require you to become physically centered. Almost every exercise will work your "core," the physical center of your body. The muscles and muscle groups of your core include your abdominal muscles (erector spinae, transversus abdominis, internal and external obliques) and the muscles contained in your buttocks, inner thighs, and lower back.

These muscle groups are not unique to the human body, but when combined they function uniquely. All movement begins with your core. These muscles enable us to stand upright and tall, which is why we are the only species on the planet that walks on two legs. It may be no coincidence that when infants develop this musculature to the extent that they are able to stand and walk, their language skills develop at light speed. This part of the body may be the epicenter of other unique abilities. Take, for instance, the sayings "I have a gut feeling" or even "He has a fire in the belly." Your center or core might just be the home of your intuition, your reason, your drive, and your will.

Along with physical core strength, a strengthening of your center may bring with it many un-expected results. Some of my clients have re-ported that their ability to reason and learn, their creativity, and their ability to conceptualize in-creased dramatically throughout their physical development. Others became more intuitive and more trusting of their instincts—their "gut" re-actions and feelings. Others have experienced that this strengthening of their center helped them follow through on projects without dis-traction for the first time. Some clients feel more ambitious and more capable; others feel virtually unstoppable. Because I have experienced all of these tangible changes from using this training system in my own life, I would contend that these inner feelings are all directly related to the development of the physical center.

Present

When you are centered, you become more pres-ent and more aware. You live more fully in the moment. As you feel more "together" in mind and body, as you become more energized and more fully activated on all levels, you will de-velop the ability to live more fully in the here and now. What is past is past, and there is noth-ing you can do to change it. The future is an open book. What you write in that book can only be written with your choices in the mo-ment. The more fully you can live and experi-ence each moment, the happier, more effective, and more successful you will become. Some people live in the past and dwell on their mis-takes and missteps. Some live in the future and fail to do today what needs to be done so they can realize their dreams later on. If you don't fol-low through with what needs to be done today, you cannot expect to realize your hopes and dreams for tomorrow. However, when you fully commit yourself to the present, a whole new world will open up to you. You will be able to give and receive more fully. You will experience improved relationships with your colleagues, as-sociates, friends, family, and loved ones. You will begin to feel an openness to the outside world and a flow to your life and surroundings. By living in the moment and using all the re-sources you possess, you will begin to live in the realm of possibility. The realm of possibility is the mind-set of "I can," "What if?" and "Yes," as opposed to a more closed perspective, whose inner dialogue sounds more like "I can't," "I could never," and "impossible."

My clients are not allowed to use phrases such as "I can't" during our training sessions. If they are in the middle of a set and I say, "Give me ten more repetitions," and they say, "I can't," I have them stop, rest, and start over until they complete the number of repetitions in the set that I requested. As their coach, I know they can finish the set, and it's my job to prove it to them. It is my job as a coach to push my clients—*and now you*—past your self-imposed limitations. We all can do more physically than we think we can, we just have to be open to the possibility. Being present and living in the realm of possi-bility will create room and space in your life. That space is precisely what will provide you with a sense of the limitless opportunities that await you.

Balance

By following the Body Express training system, you will soon find that your life is in balance.

You will feel a certain harmony, a place where your interests, obligations, and responsibilities all have their own place in your life. This sense of balance is important in helping us build a structure that will balance our personal needs, careers, families, and time. With patience and effort, you can achieve this balance.

The Power Tools

The Body Express Makeover was specifically designed to aid and develop these tools. You won't simply be going through an exercise routine. You will bring mindfulness to this physical activity and create a closer working relationship between your mental and physical functions. You will be more physically active and in so doing will be more activated on the mental, emotional, and spiritual levels. When you perform your aerobic activities, you will reduce stress, provide yourself with positive feelings of well-being and happiness, and become rejuvenated and energized. When you use the Body Express strength training programs, you will work multiple muscle groups simultaneously, and they will require you to become more present. The complexity of the movements will require you to look inward to remain centered and balanced.

Essentially, these qualities are the cornerstones for success in anything you choose to do in life. Each and every day, you will have the opportunity to develop them, but you must appreciate them enough to note and honor them. The more you note, the more you write down in your journal, the more you become consciously aware, the sooner you will attain your goals. These results are precisely what will motivate you to exercise tomorrow and the day after. You will soon feel a need to do so because the alternative (not exercising) will have absolutely no appeal. Each time you feel like using an excuse not to exercise or feel as though you are not seeing enough of a change in your body, just read through your journal and rediscover the results you have already achieved. You will come to crave these results. Feeling them will become a necessity. It will then become a reflex, a "must-do" portion of your day that gives your life quality and meaning. As soon as this is established as your new lifestyle, you will discover that you have reached, or come very close to, your ultimate goal.

Again, you *will* experience quick results with the Body Express training system. Every time you exercise during the first six weeks, I would like you to make some quick notations in your journal for that day. You should be aware of any changes or improvements, whether subtle or not, in the connection between mind and body, any shift toward a more positive outlook, feelings of stress relief, your state of happiness and well-being. Assess your energy level, your feelings of vitality, your level of mental clarity, how centered you feel, and the sense of balance in your life. If you notice it, it is worthy of mention. Write it down. For additional support, go to www.bodyexpressmakeover.com.

CHAPTER THREE

THE BODY EXPRESS

With your goals now firmly established, it is essential to understand the big picture and how all the components of the Body Express work in unison to help you accomplish your fitness goals. Again, this is a phase of contemplation, discovery, and reflection. This chapter will provide you with a frame of reference and information so that you can create an overview of the program you will utilize to achieve your goals. I will do my best to steer you in the right direction so you can make the changes in your lifestyle that you would like to.

Right now you may still be contemplating a change. You may want to change your body and lifestyle, but you may be asking yourself what are the steps that you need to take. How can you get from point A to point Z in the shortest amount of time? These are questions that will be answered in this chapter.

This chapter is about developing a strategy. In doing so, you will conquer the next phase of change, which is preparation. Believe me, I have been where you are right now. I understand your concerns and the fact that past failures may discourage you. Let go of them and open yourself to the realm of possibility. I don't care how far away you are from your ultimate goal; if it is realistic, it is attainable. I have helped find effective solutions and strategies for people of all shapes and sizes for twenty years now, and there is always a solution. You will save a lot of time by developing an effective strategy.

Exercise Works

We know that exercise works as a strategy for losing fat, weight, and inches. By increasing your level of activity, you *will* reduce body fat. When you expend energy, your body requires fuel for power. This fuel comes from the food you eat. Our fat cells act as a fuel storage system, and when we tap into this reserve tank, we lose fat.

However, if you eat so much that you never tap into your "reserve tank" of fuel, you may never call upon stored fat to power your activity. Exercise can be an effective fat fighter only if it is linked to a sound nutritional program. When you create a balanced nutritional plan and combine it with an effective activity strategy, you can structure both to reach your goal.

How Does the Body Express Makeover Work?

You can change your body quickly and forever by using this training system. It is very simple. It's simple because there are really only three ways you can change your level of fitness and improve the way you look. All of us know at least one person who has lost weight and dramatically improved the way he or she looks and feels. Think about all the people you know who have lost weight, reduced the amount of fat on their bodies, or have gotten into terrific physical condition. What did they do? If you were to interview thousands of people who successfully changed their bodies, you would discover that they have one of three things in common.

All those who have ever lost fat or inches have altered their diet, increased their activity level, or done a combination of the two. If they altered their diet, most likely they reduced the number of calories they took in and/or changed the foods they were eating, resulting in weight loss. If they increased their exercise or activity level, they simply expended more calories than they took in and therefore lost weight. However, if they did some combination of the two, they most likely lost weight and probably did so quickly. *To change your body quickly, you must do both.* Not only must you improve your eating habits and increase your activity level; you must have a winning strategy for both.

You can reduce or alter your caloric intake, you can burn off calories through exercise, or both. That's it—changing your body is really that simple! You can analyze it or pretend that there is some magic potion that will be the answer. The simple truth is that you can change the way you look only by watching what goes from your plate into your mouth and by working up a sweat. If you really want to improve your appearance—and do it quickly—the Body Express Makeover is your surest road to success.

Over the years, I have experimented on both my clients and myself. I have discovered innovative approaches that I have thoroughly developed in my training practice, and I have refined this process into a science. For instance, if an actor comes to me and needs to look a certain way in a certain number of weeks, I provide him with a road map to reach that goal. I then guide him through the process, step by step, so he hits his goal on time.

I recently helped one actor gain close to 12 pounds of muscle mass for his next movie project in just three weeks. A singer lost 10 pounds overall and 3 inches from her waist in less than four weeks before she went on tour. When I trained the contestants on *Extreme Makeover* for just two weeks, they experienced miraculous physical changes. It takes only a small window of time to make dramatic improvements to your body if you have the right formula. That's what I want to give you.

The proper nutrition, aerobic, and strength strategies are the keys to your success. There have been many books devoted to each of these topics. There is enough information available on weight training, aerobic and cardiovascular work, and various diets to fill entire libraries. In this wealth of available information, there are many viewpoints and often conflicting opinions as to which strategies are the most effective. The problem with much of this information is that there is no complete system in place, and many times there is not a lengthy track record of success. A book on nutrition may contain few, if any, exercise guidelines. On the flip side, an exercise book may not provide you with a sound nutritional strategy. I have developed the most effective and efficient training system to achieve all your fitness goals that is complete with effective strategies for weight training, aerobic training, and nutrition. This system has a track record of success for close to twenty years. I am confident that with this book you will be armed with the latest, most cutting-edge information you will need to reach your desired fitness goals.

Nutrition

As I have stated, you need a nutritional strategy that will support you in reaching your goals. This is an essential part of your makeover. The speed of your makeover will largely depend upon how well you can stick to a new way of eating that supports the changes you are trying to make. You could literally spend the rest of your life trying all the fad diets that are available to you, but, in truth, you would probably end up right where you are now: searching for answers. Diets don't work. I know you've heard it before, and it's true. Only a sound nutrition strategy that you adopt for life will work.

I will guide you through the minefield of what doesn't work and show you what has been proven to work. I will help you tailor the nutritional program that will work best for you. As soon as you begin to eat as I suggest, you will quickly see results in the mirror. You will feel your energy levels soar to new heights. In the next chapter, I will lay out a complete nutrition strategy for you. I recently had a new client who met with me for a consultation. During that consultation, I advised her on how she should be eating. Her first comment was "I'm going to starve." We had our first training session one week later because I had gone out of town. She came into my office excited and happy. She explained to me that she had already lost 3 pounds

in one week just by changing her diet and had never felt hungry or felt deprived. Not once.

While your nutritional plan will help your body release the extra body fat you are carrying, you will enhance the results even more by adding a second component to your program: aerobic activity.

Aerobic Activity

Aerobic activity—any physical activity that elevates your heart rate for a certain amount of time—will help you to burn off excess calories and stored fat. In addition to improving your strength and endurance and strengthening your heart muscle, aerobic activity is key to providing you with a longer life. Aerobic activity is the greatest pathway to burning off the stored fat that covers your muscles and to looking the way you want to look. Not only will the correct aerobic strategy improve your aesthetic appearance, it is directly linked to how good you feel, both physically and mentally. By implementing a winning nutritional and aerobic strategy, you will eliminate a great deal of the body fat you are carrying.

Strength Training

Strength training is the third ingredient in your transformation. Strength training has the greatest ability to transform your aesthetic appearance. It shapes and tones your muscles, creates symmetry, and raises your metabolism. A lot of women shy away from strength training because they are afraid they will get bulky. That is a fallacy. As long as the strength training routine is the right routine for a female body in terms of exercises, sets, and repetitions, you will not bulk up. You can rest assured that the 10-, 20-, and 30-minute Body Express Strength Training routines I developed are the right routines for a female physique. My female clients' bodies will attest to that. It is important to understand that men have testosterone in levels that women do not. For this reason, it's very difficult for the female body to put on too much muscle. The female body does not produce enough muscle-building testosterone to bulk up if trained properly. It may seem that way at first, but only because you will typically increase lean muscle mass fiber faster than you reduce your body fat percentage. The illusion is that you are bulking up, when in truth you are just toning and sculpting your muscles. Once you begin reducing the layer of body fat that is covering your muscles, you will see the muscle tone and begin to lose inches. You have to give your body a chance to catch up to the process.

Strength training will not make you muscle-bound, restrict your motion, or turn to fat. These are all myths. Strength training will tone, sculpt, and define your muscles, creating greater muscle density. This, in turn, will help your body eliminate that layer of body fat and ultimately help you attain your dream body.

The goal of strength training is to create beautiful, elongated, symmetrical muscles throughout your body. In essence, the goal is to create *density* in the musculature, not mass. There is a great difference between density and mass. Mass refers to how big a particular muscle is, whereas density refers to the amount and number of fibers within the muscle. The secret of strength training is in the density, not the size, of the muscle.

Physical training has been around for centuries. All popular forms of exercise, such as yoga, strength training, Pilates, and martial arts, have a history that goes back hundreds, if not thousands, of years. Weight-training systems such as the ones pioneered by Charles Atlas and Jack LaLanne have also been around for years and have undergone an amazing evolution of scientific precision. My Body Express Makeover workouts combine all of these practices, philosophies, and strategies into one cohesive, effective, and time-efficient routine.

These exercise routines are unique and revolutionary total-body workouts that are scientifically designed to warm up, strengthen, and then stretch each muscle group of your body. This system is a hybrid of exercise disciplines that uses complex movements combining martial arts stances and kicks, yoga postures, Pilates techniques, and core strengthening—all done simultaneously. With each exercise you will be working at least two or more muscle groups and every exercise routine is a total-body workout.

This revolutionary workout system is the ultimate in time efficiency and is designed to fit into any schedule, no matter how hectic. These exercises, which are designed to be done within ten-, twenty-, and thirty-minute windows, will provide you with a complete total-body workout that can be done in your office or hotel room, at home, or in the gym.

Putting All Three Strategies Together

In my opinion, weight loss and weight management are 70 percent dependent on sound nutrition and cardiovascular exercise. The other 30 percent is in strength training to add lean muscle mass to the body and keep it metabolically actiye to burn fuel efficiently. However, all three components are necessary for a complete transformation system. Through strength training, you will be sculpting and toning your muscles—adding lean muscle mass and decreasing your body fat percentage. By implementing a sound nutritional program, you will be feeding lean muscle and burning off fat. By engaging in aerobic exercise, you will burn excess calories and body fat, improve your circulation, strengthen your heart, increase your endurance, reduce your stress level, and increase your energy level and mental clarity; most important, you will be using stored fat to fuel your activity. When all three of these elements are in place, there is nothing—*absolutely nothing*—that can prevent you from attaining your ultimate goal.

If you are just beginning an exercise regimen, use the next three chapters as if they were a one-on-one session with me, your personal transformation coach. In the next three chapters you will learn the philosophy and the scientific principles that will be the basis of your transformation. If you have been exercising for several years, the next three chapters will be equally valuable, perhaps even more so. No matter how much you think you might know about the subject, keep an open mind. You may just pick up a few precious gems that will take your fitness level to even greater heights, and for the latest information on health and fitness, go to www.bodyexpressmakeover.com.

CHAPTER FOUR

FAT-BLASTING NUTRITION

No matter what your goal, it is essential to create a strategy for a new way of eating. The key to reducing body fat, and maintaining that loss, is mastering the termination stage of change. Mastering your diet will enable you (and others) to see your newly toned and sculpted muscles and will dramatically improve your overall health.

Did you know that in a recent study it was found that junk food (chips, soda, candy) makes up approximately one third of the total calories in the average American's diet? We are the most obese nation in the Western world, yet we have access to the highest quality of fresh food. Why do you think that is? The answer is very simple: we are simply making the wrong food choices. It's time to take responsibility for what we put in our mouths each and every day.

Creating a nutrition program that works may have been confusing in the past. However, I am going to simplify how you should eat so there will be no more confusion. I am going to give you the tools that will empower you to make healthier choices. I'm talking about the kind of empowerment that comes only from a gut feeling that says, "This makes perfect sense." I have been successful in creating a winning eating strategy for my clients, and with my "fat-blasting" nutritional strategy, you will get the results you are looking for quickly and without feeling deprived or hungry. You will dis-cover the exact nutritional balance that you can easily adhere to for the rest of your life. This nutritional strategy can easily be incorporated into your life with a little planning and trust in the program. You will have to trust that I know what works when it comes to weight loss and weight management.

Confusion

There is a wealth of information available on dieting and weight loss, most of which touts claims of "get thin quickly" while you "eat whatever you want." These are gimmicks. There is simply too much information to sort through, too many different programs to experiment with, and far too many potential paths that will result in a weight loss roller-coaster ride. There are so many philosophies and products vying for your weight loss dollar that it is difficult to know what to pay attention to and what to dis-regard. Advertising is one of the main culprits that hinders our ability to make an informed decision.

The next time you are in the checkout line

at the grocery store, pick up any women's magazine and flip through its pages. You will see the almost schizophrenic conundrum we are all facing. We are bombarded with conflicting messages. One article or ad entices us into eating; the next encourages us to lose weight, sometimes even on the same page. Turn on your TV, and you will see a slick commercial for your favorite fast-food restaurant followed by another commercial for some weight loss pill. Radio advertising is even more extreme. Consume . . . lose . . . consume . . . lose. Does this sound vaguely familiar to you? Is it any wonder that this is precisely the nutritional cycle by which most of us live? When we decide to go on a diet, the plan is to restrict our eating. Often we then rationalize having a "treat" or giving ourselves permission to "splurge" because we will be depriving ourselves the next day. Think about when you go on a diet. How do you celebrate when you reach your weight goal? If you are like most people, you probably slowly begin to consume the very foods that made you gain the weight in the first place, the very foods you eliminated from your diet to lose weight! Most often that means starchy carbohydrates such as bread, pasta, potatoes, rice, sugar, and processed foods. In a short time you are back where you started, having gained back the weight you lost and many times, more. Let's get something straight: *fad diets do not work!* They never have, and they never will. That said, let's find out what does work.

The Fat-Blasting Nutrition strategy has four basic principles. You may have seen or heard about some of these principles, but when all of them are applied simultaneously, losing excess body fat becomes simple and fast. These four steps are the building blocks of a healthy diet, and, with a little planning, they are easy to incorporate into your lifestyle. My clients who follow these four principles, along with my cardio suggestions and my 2-in-1 strength training routines, lose weight and lose it quickly. They are able to sculpt, tone, shape, and build lean muscle efficiently and effectively—and, most important, maintain it.

These are the principles of Fat-Blasting Nutrition. Now let's learn why this eating strategy works.

Searching for What Works

Without question, creating a nutritional game plan you can live with is the single most important factor in creating and maintaining a

---

THE FOUR PRINCIPLES

Principle 1:
Use the 40:30:30 ratio for each meal: 40 percent carbohydrate, 30 percent protein, 30 percent fat. Eat a little protein with each meal.

Principle 2:
Eat five small meals or snacks per day. Eat a small meal every 2½ to 3 hours. Portion control and moderation are key.

Principle 3:
Choose low glycemic carbohydrates over high glycemic carbohydrates. Eat carbohydrates strategically, and increase your consumption of high-fiber foods.

Principle 4:
Choose fresh produce and lean meats. Reduce your consumption of processed and high-sugar foods.

---

better-looking body. I have spent many years researching and experimenting with various diet plans. I've tried every diet plan imaginable. I have consulted with top nutritionists, which has led me to design a nutrition plan that is simple, easy to follow, and extremely effective. It has helped my clients to look and feel the best they could.

Clarifying Your Weight Loss Goal

The first test of any nutritional program is to determine if it will help you reach and maintain your desired weight goal throughout your life. Let's get really specific about weight loss. Your weight on the scale has nothing to do with how you look. If you feel as though you are too heavy, the weight you would like to lose is really the *body fat* you want to lose. Most of our body weight is made up of water, and many of the fad diets are simply diuretics that cannibalize muscle tissue. After being on a fad diet for a week or two, you may have lost some "weight" when you look at the scale, but that weight was most likely just water weight along with some lean muscle mass, which your body cannibalized for energy. If you finally found a diet or nutritional strategy that would help you shed unwanted pounds easily, without feeling deprived or hungry, one that you could adhere to for life, what would that mean to you? Ponder that thought for a moment, because today is the day for that discovery.

Fat-Blasting Nutrition

First, you will create the proper balance between carbohydrates, protein, and fats and understand why eating a little protein with each meal is important. Second, you will learn why you should eat five small meals or snacks per day and mon-itor your portions. Third, you will learn to distinguish between high and low glycemic carbohydrates and how to eat them strategically. Fourth, you will reduce your intake of processed foods and eat fresh, healthy, fiber-rich foods. This four-step Fat-Blasting Nutrition strategy is your road map to the *you* you are looking to create and a lifestyle that will support permanent weight management.

PRINCIPLE 1: USE THE 40:30:30 RATIO FOR EACH MEAL

The first principle of creating a successful nutritional program is to determine what to eat and in what proportion. It is vitally important to create the proper ratio of protein, carbohydrates, and fat in each meal or snack. Over the last ten years, there have been many innovations in nutritional science. Many of these advances have created contradictions and rifts within the scientific community. Diet books that advise reducing your carbohydrate intake to a minimum and eating a high-protein diet have popularized many of these new innovations.

While increased protein intake is beneficial and important, high-protein diets are extreme and unrealistic in the long term, especially for individuals with busy lifestyles. It typically takes more time to prepare foods and meals that are high in protein than to reach for a bag of chips or a candy bar. Essentially these diets prescribe a high-protein diet to elicit a certain hormonal response that facilitates rapid weight loss by putting the body into a state of ketosis. Ketosis is an abnormal increase of acidic biochemicals in the blood and urine and a sign that the metabolism is impaired. These acidic biochemicals are produced when there isn't enough glucose in the bloodstream. High levels of ketones make blood abnormally acidic. Does that sound healthy to you?

Many people on high-protein diets initially see rapid weight loss due to the body being shocked into doing so, but eventually they reach a plateau. For the most part, people on high-protein diets cannot sustain this way of eating for longer than three to six months. Then what? They go back to their old way of eating and end up where they started, or worse. There are three serious problems with high-protein diets. First, as I mentioned, they are hard to maintain. Second, they are typically high in saturated fat, which contributes to clogged arteries and an increased risk of heart attacks. Last, there are not enough long-term studies to prove that eating a high-protein diet is safe. Long-term studies have shown that people on a *higher-protein* diet—not a high-protein diet that dramatically reduces carbohydrates—have a greater success rate in reducing body fat and maintaining that weight loss in the long term. I tell you this because I have seen it hundreds of times with my own clients.

So what is the answer? After experimenting with every diet under the sun, I have found that a *higher-protein* diet works very well for approximately 75 percent of the population for weight reduction and weight management. The diet philosophy I'm referring to is "The Zone" by Dr. Barry Sears. His philosophy makes sense because it prescribes that 40 percent of your diet should come from low to moderate glycemic carbohydrates such as most fruits and vegetables, 30 percent from lean sources of protein, and 30 percent from "good" fats. This is a balanced, realistic nutrition plan that one can easily adhere to for life. It's how I instruct my clients to eat, and on average they experience a consistent weight loss of 2 pounds of body fat per week. I know there are some high-protein diets that claim 8 to 13 pounds of weight loss without exercise in the first two weeks. I won't dwell on this claim other than to say that even if someone did lose that amount of weight, not all of it would be from fat loss, and it would definitely be the exception to the rule, not the norm.

Body fat reduction is all about eating in a way that safely manipulates one's hormonal response to insulin. More specifically, it's about using food in combinations that limit the secretion of insulin. The main function of insulin is to sweep up "extra" or unused carbohydrates in the bloodstream and store them as fat for later use. Not only that, but increased insulin levels inhibit the body's ability to release the stored fat. What does that mean? It means that it becomes virtually impossible to utilize stored body fat for energy. In general terms, the premise of a *higher-protein* diet is to reduce the secretion of insulin by reducing the amount of high glycemic carbohydrates you eat and in what combinations you eat them.

What we are really talking about here is a hormonal response to the foods you eat. We are talking specifically about insulin and the amount of it that is released into the bloodstream. *The greater the quantity of insulin released, the more calories are stored as fat and the less fat the body releases for energy usage.*

Insulin is released into the bloodstream in response to glucose, which is essentially sugar. Any carbohydrate, after being digested, breaks down into its basic chemical compound, glucose. That means that any carbohydrate, whether it be table sugar, fruit, bread, pasta, rice, or a starchy vegetable such as a potato, will eventually be turned into glucose by the time it enters your bloodstream. The greater the quantity of glucose in your bloodstream, the more insulin is secreted. When a certain level of glucose is detected in your bloodstream, your body secretes insulin to remove the excess.

Our goal here is to find ways to slow down the rate of glucose absorption. The slower the rate of absorption of a carbohydrate, the less apt the body is to store it as fat. The three factors that determine the rate of absorption of a particular food are the type of carbohydrate, the fiber content, and the fat content. We refer to this as the glycemic index (absorption rate). We want to eat primarily low- to moderate-glycemic-index carbohydrates, such as *most* fruits and vegetables, which also happen to be high in fiber. High-glycemic-index foods such as processed bread, baked goods, candy, chips, potatoes, rice, and pasta raise insulin levels and can inhibit weight loss. Pasta and rice are the exception if they are consumed in the right proportion and combined with the right food, such as a lean protein source.

Some carbohydrates are more complex than others and have a longer molecular chain. Therefore, the digestive process is required to work harder to break them down into their basic material (glucose or sugar) because of the increase in fiber. Fiber and fat both help slow down the digestive process and help satiate us faster. The result is that we feel fuller for longer periods of time and typically reduce the amount of calories we ingest because we feel full.

Dr. Barry Sears, in his book *The Zone,* popularized the notion of eating more low- to moderate-glycemic-index carbohydrates and more lean protein to facilitate weight loss, opti-mize energy levels, and reduce the chance of developing adult-onset diseases. Remember, at the beginning of the chapter I said that a successful nutrition strategy needs to support your weight loss efforts and be realistic for life. The 40:30:30 ratio is a very realistic, balanced, healthy diet that you can adhere to for life. Today the term "glycemic index" has entered in the lexicon of our diet vocabulary. Essentially, the glycemic index rates all carbohydrates according to their complexity, rate of absorption, and their immediate effect on blood sugar. The higher the rating, the more insulin is secreted. Here is how it works. Foods that have a high GI rating are absorbed and digested by the body very quickly, causing dramatic fluctuations in blood-sugar levels, thus raising insulin levels. Low GI foods have the opposite effect and greatly lower and control glucose and lipid levels. Low GI foods help to control and manage weight because they satiate you for a longer period of time and delay hunger. In doing so, low GI foods will also aid you in reducing caloric intake without your feeling deprived.

Eating Protein with Each Meal

Let's say you eat a simple carbohydrate, such as a piece of fruit or a candy bar. Eaten alone, it would enter your bloodstream in the form of glucose and raise your insulin level almost instantly. Proteins, such as lean cuts of meat, poultry, fish, eggs, nuts, and low-fat dairy products, take much longer to digest and are broken down into their smallest components, amino acids. Amino acids, for the most part, do not stimulate insulin secretion. Protein also requires the body to put forth a greater amount of effort for a longer period of time to digest it, which once again slows down the digestive process.

When a carbohydrate is eaten *in combination with* a protein, it becomes a new source of energy on a molecular level. So when a simple carbohydrate is eaten in combination with a lean protein source, such as a piece of cheese or a slice of turkey, that combination of foods goes through a very different digestive process than if either is eaten alone. *When you combine carbohydrates with proteins, less glucose enters the bloodstream, and it is released over a longer duration of time. This lowers your insulin level so your body can burn the carbohydrates as fuel as opposed to storing them as fat.*

Another important factor to consider is those endless cravings for sugar or carbohydrates. Eating a little protein with each meal will reduce your cravings for such foods. Let me explain. When you eat sugar or a carbohydrate alone, it raises (spikes) your insulin levels, but what goes up must come down. So when your insulin level drops, it creates a craving for more sugar or carbohydrates for immediate energy and to get "high" again, because now you are feeling tired and lethargic. Sounds like an addiction, right? It's something to think about. However, when you eat a little protein with each meal, which forces the secretion of glucagon (the hormone that stimulates insulin secretion), your insulin level balances out so your body doesn't go through the insulin roller-coaster ride. The result is that you have a sustained, well-balanced energy level throughout the day instead of that tired, lethargic feeling you may usually experience around midafternoon.

The premise behind a *higher-protein* diet is that it's not the protein or fat in our daily diet that is causing the obesity epidemic, it is the excess of high glycemic carbohydrates and carbohydrates eaten alone and in excess that create and store fat. In other words, lean sources of protein and good fats will not make you fat if they are eaten in the proper proportion. Fat does not induce a secretion of insulin. Do you remember the low-fat craze that swept through our country not so long ago? Every major food manufacturer jumped on the bandwagon and made low-fat versions of almost every food product. What happened? We got fatter, not thinner! We ended up eating more of those low-fat foods because they didn't fill us up due to the reduced fat content and the fact that they were high in sugar and carbohydrates. Consider this: an entire chicken breast has approximately 300 calories; a small Snickers bar has approximately 275 calories. The chicken breast does not require the secretion of insulin, but the Snickers bar does. As a consequence, when eating the Snickers bar there is a greater chance your body will store these calories in your fat cells; eating the chicken breast will not.

Creating the Proper Nutritional Balance

I want you to eat some protein with each and every meal. All of my clients have had great success using a higher-protein diet. Not a *high-protein* diet, but a *higher-protein* diet. As you have read, there is a big distinction between the two. Simply put, eating a diet that is *higher* in protein helps balance out the hormonal release of insulin and is an integral part of your healthy, balanced nutritional plan. This is worth repeating: Another reason a higher-protein diet works for weight loss and weight management is that by eating fewer carbohydrates and more lean protein and good fats, we feel fuller faster so we ingest less calories per meal. There is one universal deduction in light of all the scientific research studies that have come out: Weight loss is all about calories in and calories out. If you reduce your caloric intake, you will reduce your body fat percentage.

In each of your many meals or snacks, I suggest creating a balance of protein, carbohydrates, and fat of 40 percent carbohydrate, 30 percent protein, and 30 percent fat. The easiest way to make this new nutritional program work is to use the "eyeball" method and determine what your plate should look like. This is the simple part. When you look at your plate, one third of your meal should be made up of a lean protein source such as fish, tofu, chicken, or lamb. The remaining two thirds of your plate should be made up of low to moderate glycemic carbohydrates, primarily from vegetables and fruits. It's that simple.

As for the type of fat you want in your diet, it is important to choose "good" fats versus "bad" ones. In Dr. Sears's words, "We want to use fat to burn fat." Saturated fats and trans fats (artificial fats) are the bad fats that cause high cholesterol, clogged arteries, and heart disease. Trans fats come from the hydrogenated oils in our time-saving invention: processed foods. This is why your protein sources should always be lean cuts of meat and poultry and you should rely on low-fat dairy products. Monounsaturated fats are the good fats that can be found in olive oil, canola oil, omega-3 fatty acids (in fish and fish oil), most nuts, and avocados. When cooking, you can use butter and certain oils to

flavor your food as long as you do so in moderation and not in excess.

By balancing your meals and snacks in this proportion, you will be effectively balancing all the hormones that are at work during the digestion process, and you will eliminate those insulin spikes. My nutritional game plan will work in more ways than one to alleviate that cycle of insulin peaks and valleys. First, a consistent balance of food ratios will provide a stable blood sugar level, which will lower your insulin levels and raise your glucagon and HGH (human growth hormone) levels. It will eliminate much of the excess cortisol (stress hormone) from your blood. By eating high-quality lean proteins, low to moderate glycemic carbohydrates, and healthy fats, you will teach your body to process food and burn calories more efficiently. In just a few weeks you will have successfully trained your body to utilize body fat as your primary fuel source.

Of course, there are exceptions to every rule. The ratio of 40 percent carbohydrate, 30 percent protein, and 30 percent fat is the best nutrition plan for approximately 75 percent of the population. Approximately 25 percent of the population, due to their genetic makeup, ancestry, and several other determinates, actually control weight gain and energy levels better on a higher-carbohydrate diet. However, these are also the people who don't need to lose weight (body fat), because they naturally possess a very fast metabolism.

PRINCIPLE 2: EATING FIVE SMALL MEALS OR SNACKS PER DAY

The second principle of weight loss and weight management requires you to outthink your body. You were born with a whole set of innate survival tools. Many of our body's survival tools and mechanisms rely on stored fat. Way back when, we were hunters and gatherers, and because of this our food intake tended to be inconsistent. Coaxing your most primitive survival mechanisms into releasing your stored fat will require some conscious planning on your part. Eating *five small meals or snacks* every 2½ to 3 hours every day for the rest of your life is a very important component of permanent weight management. Breakfast, lunch, and dinner were structured for us so that we could farm, hunt, fight wars, and work in offices and manufacturing plants—however, eating three large meals per day is not how our bodies want to be fed.

All of us were born with a starvation protection device, and it is hardwired into our cells to ensure our survival. If you go too long between meals, this primitive survival instinct does not know that food is as close as the refrigerator or the next convenience store. Your body simply thinks it is starving. Consequently, it will expend only a minimal amount of energy to fuel the most basic bodily functions and store the rest as fat. When you finally get around to eating again, your body (which is in survival mode) will store much of that food in your fat cells for later use. To coax your body into releasing this stored fat, you must remove its fear of famine. Your starvation protection mechanism must never be allowed to go into action. Your body must never think it is being starved. If you can relax the starvation protection mechanism, you will have great success. If you do not, your efforts will be futile.

Timing, as they say, is everything. The quickest way to activate your natural fat-burning ability centers on the timing of your meals. Your starvation protection mechanism can be lulled into a sense of security only if it is reassured that your body is being fed. Instead of eating the traditional three big meals, I want you to eat *five smaller meals or snacks* throughout the day.

Again, this is about activating your natural body fat–burning furnace. It is essential that you eat your first meal or snack within sixty minutes of waking up and a small meal or snack every 2½ to 3 hours. Without a doubt, breakfast is the most important meal of the day. Many of us go without breakfast and, as a result, rob ourselves of the most fundamental step to jumpstart our metabolism into high gear. After a full night of rest and many hours without food, the body needs to be fueled as soon as possible. When we go without this vital meal, we are robbing ourselves of the opportunity to fuel the furnace of our metabolism. The only exception is if you are going to do an aerobic workout immediately upon waking. Then you can wait until after you exercise because you will be utilizing primarily your fat stores as an energy source, which is what we want to do.

The objective is to speed up your metabolism to its highest possible level, burning all the fuel you put into the furnace quickly and completely. When you eat a small meal shortly after waking, you jump-start your metabolism. After 2½ to 3 hours, your body will have used up that fuel and you will need to replenish your fuel source. I can't say it often enough: to keep your metabolism on its highest setting, eat *five small meals or snacks* throughout the day.

If you eat five small meals or snacks throughout the day and at roughly the same time each day, your body will soon get into a new rhythm of eating. In essence, it will begin to trust that it will be fed regularly. It will begin to trust that it does not have to lock down what is held in storage within your fat cells, and it will begin to release body fat naturally. Your body will adjust so that it expends what you eat for fuel rather than conserve or store away nutrients for later use. This is the process of speeding up your metabolism.

Obstacles

It does not seem as though this should be a difficult proposition, but eating this many times and at roughly the same times every day takes planning. The largest obstacle you will face is time. It takes time to prepare for this new way of eating. You will have scheduling conflicts. Your day might not go as planned. You may have to take your lunch to work with you or keep some healthy snacks in your briefcase. You may have to force yourself to take breaks so that you can have light snacks. I highly recommend keeping foods such as fruit, nuts, protein bars, or beef jerky in your car. I also suggest taking a small cooler to work with you so that you can keep things such as tuna, chicken, sliced cheese or turkey, cottage cheese, and cut-up veggies in your office. It takes a little planning at first, but it will soon become second nature and be well worth the effort.

We are all in a hurry. Our hurried lifestyle is a major part of the obesity problem in this country. We are busier now than ever before. We spend less time with our loved ones and on our hobbies or recreational activities. Do you know that in some countries in Europe it is normal to take a siesta after lunch? When was the last time you took a siesta after lunch? Many European countries also take longer vacations, and many companies even shut down for periods of time so their workers can take their vacations. Unfortunately, most large U.S. companies are more interested in the almighty dollar than the health of their employees, which is why you need to be proactive when it comes to your health.

For those of you who are time-challenged, I strongly recommend that you remind yourself of this fact: when embarking on a fitness regimen, it is vital to take time for yourself when it comes to eating and exercising. To successfully absorb the notion of "making time" and incorporate it into your lifestyle, you must take the necessary steps to ensure that food is ready and available when you need it. Because most of us are on the go and "don't have time," when we finally get around to eating, we are so hungry that we choose the quickest remedy: fast food.

There is no surer way to increase your body fat percentage than to make fast food a mainstay of your diet. Remember the documentary film *Super Size Me,* about the guy who ate just McDonald's food for thirty days? After twenty-one days, his doctors asked him to quit because he was putting his life in jeopardy! The fast-food industry is a multibillion-dollar industry. Granted, many of the fast-food chains are now offering healthier food choices, which *is* a step in the right direction. On the West Coast we have several fast-service chains like Koo Koo Roo, El Pollo Loco, and Baja Fresh that offer healthier food choices such as rotisserie or grilled chicken, steamed vegetables, and salads. I realize that eating at fast-food restaurants cannot always be avoided due to your busy schedule, but the key is to make healthier food choices. Instead of a burger, fries, and a Coke, why not have a chicken sandwich (removing the top piece of bread) with a side salad and iced tea? The average American eats three hamburgers and four orders of fries every week. I'm not saying never have a burger and fries. What I am saying is to lose body fat, you need to eat in a way that supports that goal more consistently.

I know that time is an issue for most of you, but do your best to sit down to eat your meals and snacks. When we eat on the run or while watching television, eating becomes an unconscious activity. It isn't that the food isn't as beneficial, but psychologically the meal is not as fulfilling as it could be if you were giving it your complete attention. An example of this phenomenon is the family dinner. Not so long ago, most families ate their evening meal together each night at a designated time. The most recent studies from the Centers for Disease Control and Prevention have shown that 90 percent of children who almost always eat a traditional dinner at home with other family members are not overweight and are much leaner than children who eat dinner without that family structure. The same studies have shown that this is also true for adults with or without children. Making time to truly enjoy your food and the people who are important to you not only allows you to appreciate a meal more but also provides you with an opportunity to spend quality time with friends and loved ones. This is another benefit of living a healthier lifestyle—spending more quality time with loved ones. I strongly recommend that you attempt to make a habit of eating a traditional evening meal.

Portion Control

The supersize . . . seconds . . . the buffet . . . all you can eat . . . As a nation, we are blessed with bounty. However, our culture also fosters overconsumption. We need to think of food as a fuel or as a drug that regulates hormone levels to prevent overeating. The key is to strike a balance between enough and too much, which is essential when it comes to the delicate balance of shutting down your starvation mechanism. Portion control involves creating a balance where you eat enough food to prevent the starvation protection mechanism from becoming activated but not enough that the "extra" food is stored within your fat cells.

Enough and Too Much

You do not need a lot of food at any one meal or snack. Your stomach is a relatively small organ containing water, enzymes, acids, and compounds that break down your food into molecular particles. Your body is simply not equipped to efficiently consume a Thanksgiving-sized meal on a daily basis. Your many small meals or snacks should be just that—small.

I'm not big on measuring food, for two reasons. First, I think it's unrealistic to have to stop every time you need to eat and measure your food. Second, measuring food does not necessarily support behavior modification and therefore does not support long-term weight management. You can't just pull out a scale at a restaurant or dinner party or when you're traveling. What you can do is use the eyeball method. It's a tried-and-true method that has been around for years. **A portion of protein or car-**

DAILY CALORIE CHART

The charts below represent an estimate of how many calories you can eat each day and still lose weight. These are estimates and the actual calories you need may vary depending on your age, gender, and level of physical activity.

MALES

Weight	Ages 20–30	Ages 31–50	Ages 50+
130–155 lbs.	1600–1800 Kcals	1500–1650 Kcals	1400 Kcals
156–195 lbs.	1800–2000 Kcals	1650–1800 Kcals	1500–1600 Kcals
196–250 lbs.	2000–2200 Kcals	1800–2000 Kcals	1600–1800 Kcals

FEMALES

Weight	Ages 20–30	Ages 31–50	Ages 50+
130–155 lbs.	1300–1450 Kcals	1400 Kcals	1250–1400 Kcals
156–195 lbs.	1500–1700 Kcals	1400–1550 Kcals	1400–1600 Kcals
196–250 lbs.	1800–2000 Kcals	1650–1800 Kcals	1600 Kcals

bohydrates at a meal is typically the size of your open palm. A snack-sized portion of cheese would be the size of your finger; a handful of nuts is ten to twelve almonds. Your plate at any meal should contain 350–500 calories, consisting of one portion of a lean protein source (chicken, turkey, fish, soy products, nuts) and one to two portions of low to moderate glycemic carbohydrates in the form of high-fiber fruits and vegetables. A snack should look like a smaller version of a meal and be only 100 to 150 calories.

Once you begin to make healthier food choices, you must be careful of the carbohydrate portion of your plate. The average American eats a great many calories, up to one third, in the form of simple, starchy high glycemic carbohydrates, such as sugary foods and drinks, bread, and potatoes. I would like to make one note here. Pasta and rice have received a bad rap lately for being high glycemic carbohydrates. To the contrary, because pasta is made from durum wheat, which your body digests more slowly than white flour, most pastas, not all, if cooked al dente, are actually a low to moderate GI carbohydrate. Most types of rice fall under the category of a moderate GI carbohydrate. The problem most people face when eating pasta or rice is that their portion sizes tend to be too high, they eat these two foods too often, or they don't eat these foods strategically. I suggest a portion size of ½ to 1 cup of pasta or rice per meal and it must be eaten with some form of lean protein. These two foods should be eaten in the early part of the day and in moderation so they can be utilized and burned for energy. You can have some pasta or rice, but no more than three times per week or preferably less if weight loss is your primary goal. I'm not giving you the total green light here to indulge in pasta or rice. But you can eat them in moderation depending on your weight-loss goals and how fast you want to shed those excess pounds. The more you reduce high glycemic carbohydrates, the faster you will see results. All of us are accustomed to eating simple carbohydrates. It is part of our cultural mind-set. But to shed excess pounds, it is essential to shed our addiction to simple sugars and starchy carbohydrates. It will take some time and patience, but you will actually reeducate your taste buds to enjoy healthier foods. They say it takes twenty-eight days to break a habit, so be consistent and diligent. I promise, it will happen. It happened for me and countless clients of mine.

Choosing nutrient-rich foods that your body requires to restore your hormonal balance will not happen overnight, and it may be a little challenging at first. Do not get discouraged. After a few short weeks, your body should begin to adjust to nutrient-rich foods rather than unhealthy ones. In fact, your body may begin to react negatively to the unhealthy foods it once craved. For this reason, I suggest that you choose to prepare your food in the most natural way. The less processed, the better.

Moderation

I know what you're thinking. Am I saying that you can never eat a baked potato, a slice of bread, a piece of pie, or a Snickers bar ever again? No. I don't expect you to live a life of deprivation, because that is unrealistic. This is where things can get tricky. This is where you are going to have to be brutally honest with and accountable to yourself. This is the realm of moderation. Eating too much of the wrong foods made you gain weight and body fat. Now

I'm asking you to eat more of the right foods to lose that body fat and maintain the fat loss throughout your life. It's just not realistic to eat the wrong foods on a regular basis and still expect to lose weight.

I want you to eat foods that are high in protein, such as chicken, fish, lean cuts of beef, lamb, egg whites, and nuts. I want you to eat foods that are high in fiber, such as most fruits and vegetables and true whole grains. Please note that the wheat bread you buy at your local supermarket is typically processed in much the same way as white bread; I'm talking about whole grain bread that actually has whole grains or sprouts in it. By following these few simple suggestions, you *will* experience weight loss quickly. When you choose to eat simple sugars or starchy high glycemic carbohydrates, I ask that you eat them strategically—in moderation and in small portions, the size of your palm.

Later in the chapter, we will discuss strategic eating. Most social events, business meetings, romantic dates, and get-togethers with friends and family revolve around the consumption of food. Eating is a part of our social culture and will remain so for a long time to come. My suggestion is to occasionally eat a small bowl (½ cup) of pasta or half a baked potato. Take a couple of bites of dessert instead of eating the whole thing. Have a few fries, not a supersized portion, with your burger wrapped in lettuce rather than a bun. Other times, have a side salad or a vegetable with your burger and take one bun off. Instead of having a bag of chips, eat a handful every so often. What I'm asking you to do is to reduce how often you eat these types of foods, eat them in moderation when you do, and eat a little protein with each meal. That's not asking too much, is it?

Eating healthfully means being more aware of your food choices and, at times, making compromises. Isn't a relationship with a spouse all about compromise? Am I being unrealistic to ask this of you? We are all intelligent enough to know that a diet made up of junk food and starchy high glycemic carbohydrates is not going to support our fitness goals. So let's just admit that reducing these foods is the solution and get on with it. If you cannot reduce how often you eat these foods and eat them in moderation when you do, you will have to eliminate them from your diet completely until such time as you can eat them in moderation—if ever. There is no other magic solution. This will be the most difficult of truths to face. Let's be honest: these are the foods that made you fat. I understand that you will experience setbacks and times when you will revert back to old habits and patterns, but the key is to acknowledge them and move on. Remember, you are embarking on a new lifestyle. There will be setbacks. Your goal is to stay the course and keep moving forward despite them. Give credit to the fact that you are doing your best, and use that fact to motivate yourself to make healthier food choices. Living a healthy lifestyle is not about being perfect, it's about doing the best you can every day. It's about continually raising the bar of your own expectations of yourself so that you are happy with your choices.

PRINCIPLE 3: CHOOSE LOW GLYCEMIC CARBOHYDRATES OVER HIGH GLYCEMIC CARBOHYDRATES

There has been a lot of discussion in the media recently about reducing carbohydrate intake, but what does that mean? Many food companies and fast-food restaurants are coming out with low-carbohydrate versions of their menu offerings. Are all carbohydrates bad for you? No, they are not. Your body needs carbohydrates as much as it needs protein and fat. Your brain needs carbohydrates to function properly, and your body needs them as an energy source. You want to use your excess fat as an energy source, but that energy source can go only so far. What the diet industry has determined as "bad" carbohydrates are the ones that elicit the high insulin response because their high glycemic index causes them to enter the bloodstream quickly. "Good" or low to moderate glycemic carbohydrates do the exact opposite: they enter the bloodstream slowly and elicit a low insulin response. However, I don't like to refer to carbohydrates as "good" or "bad"; they are simply either high, moderate, or low glycemic, due to their effect on insulin.

The Glycemic Index ranks carbohydrates from 0 to 100 based on how quickly they enter the bloodstream and cause blood sugar and insulin levels to rise. The Glycemic Index chart is ranked below.

- Low glycemic carbohydrates are listed as 55 or less
- Medium or moderate glycemic carbohydrates are listed as 56 to 69
- High glycemic carbohydrates are listed as 70 and above

Listed first in the Glycemic Index Food List are low glycemic, fiber-rich carbohydrates. If you can eat from this list most of the time, you will have great success in dropping body fat and in managing your weight in the long term.

Glycemic Index Food List
Low Glycemic Food Choices

FOOD	GI
Apples	35
Artichoke hearts	50
Bananas	53
Bean sprouts	low
Black beans	30
Black-eyed peas	42
Bread (pumpernickel)	49
Broccoli	50
Brown rice	55
Buckwheat	54
Cauliflower	low
Cherries	23
Chickpeas (boiled)	33
Chocolate	49
Eggplant	low
Fruit cocktail	55
Grapes	43
Grapefruit	25
Green beans	30
Ice cream (low fat)	50
Instant noodles	47
Kidney beans (boiled)	27
Kiwis	52
Lentils (boiled)	29
Lima beans	32
Mangoes	55
Milk (skim)	32
Navy beans (boiled)	54
Oatmeal	55
Onions	low
Oranges	43
Pasta (angel hair)	45
Pasta (vermicelli)	35
Pasta (whole grain)	45
Peaches	28
Peanuts	13
Pears	35
Peppers	low
Plums	25
Romano beans	46

FOOD	GI
Soy beans (boiled)	18
Spaghetti (whole grain)	38
Special K	54
Split peas	32
Sponge cake	54
Squash	low
Strawberry	32
Sweet corn	55
Sweet potato	54
Tomatoes	38
Vegetables (green)	low
Water chestnuts	low
Yams	51
Yogurt	33
Yogurt (sugar free)	14

Moderate Glycemic Food Choices

FOOD	GI
Angel food cake	67
Apricots	57
Baked beans (canned)	68
Beets	64
Bran	60
Bread (rye)	65
Blueberry	59
Cantaloupe	65
Corn	59
Cornmeal	68
Couscous	65
Cream of Wheat	66
Gnocchi	65
Hamburger bun	61
Ice cream	61
Life cereal	66
Macaroni	64
Orange Juice	57
Pasta (refined)	65
Pineapple	66
Pinto beans (canned)	64
Pita bread (whole wheat)	58
Pizza (cheese)	60
Puffed wheat	67
Raisins	64

Rice (not instant)	56	Potato (white, boiled)	90
Rye Flour	65	Potato (white, mashed)	73
Shredded Wheat	69	PowerBar	83
Shortbread	64	Pumpkin	75
		Puffed rice	90

High Glycemic Food Choices

FOOD	GI		
		Pretzels	80
Bagel (white)	72	Rice (white, instant)	88
Bread (sourdough)	74	Rice cakes	77
Bread (white)	96	Rice Chex	90
Bread (whole wheat)	75	Rice Krispies	82
Carrots	71	Rutabagas	72
Cherios	74	Skittles	70
Coca-Cola (regular)	90	Soda	70
Cocoa Pops	77	Tofu (frozen dessert)	115
Corn chips	73	Vanilla wafers	77
Cornflakes	84	Waffles	76
Corn tortilla	70	Water crackers	72
Crispix	87	Watermelon	72
Croissant (medium)	96		
Doughnut	76		
Dried fruit	70		
English muffin	77		
Fava beans	80		
French fries	75		
Gatorade	111		
Glucose	100		
Golden Grahams	71		
Granola bar	87		
Grapenut Flakes	80		
Honey	73		
Kaiser rolls	73		
Jelly beans	80		
Linguine (thin)	79		
Mangoes	80		
Millet	71		
Papayas (medium)	82		
Parsnips	97		
Popcorn (plain)	89		
Pop-Tart (chocolate)	70		
Potato (baked)	85		
Potato (instant)	83		
Potato (red, boiled)	126		

Eating Carbohydrates Strategically

Eating carbohydrates strategically is important. This is where awareness comes into play. If you eat meals and snacks that are high in high glycemic carbohydrates early in the day, you will need to reduce your high GI carbohydrate intake dramatically later in the day. Conversely, if you know you are going out to dinner with friends or family in the evening, try to consume less high glycemic carbohydrates during the day so that you can enjoy your dinner without feeling guilty. If you intend to have dessert, be conscious of that when you order your dinner and make sure your dinner is a balanced 40:30:30 meal of lean protein and vegetables. Then, when you get the dessert, have a couple of bites and pass it around for the rest of the table to try.

As I said earlier, it is preferable to eat your high glycemic (starchy) carbohydrates earlier in the day and taper them off throughout the day.

In other words, your last meal of the day should come primarily from lean protein sources, vegetables, and fruit. Why is this important? You expend energy (calories) throughout each day just by being in motion. If you eat your starchy carbohydrates before 1 P.M., you allow yourself time to burn those high glycemic carbohydrate calories as fuel. However, if you eat them late in the day, when you are typically less active, you are less likely to burn off those calories and more apt to store them as fat.

Another time you want to eat your high glycemic carbohydrates is immediately following an exercise session. Your body has a window of thirty to forty-five minutes post exercise to maximize glycogen replenishment and utilize those carbohydrates optimally. If you do your exercise sessions in the evenings, my suggestion is to ingest only low to moderate glycemic carbohydrate late in the day after a workout.

Eating carbohydrates strategically is a very important component of this program. All it takes is a little awareness and foresight to salvage any poor eating day or even to rescue it. Remember, it's your state of mind that makes all the difference. Don't give in to the impulse to eat high glycemic carbohydrates when you can consciously make a healthier choice. That is self-defeating behavior, and I don't know if you remember, but we checked that behavior at the door a long time ago. Remember: not succeeding is *not an option.*

PRINCIPLE 4: CHOOSE FRESH PRODUCE AND LEAN MEATS

Let's examine the nutrients contained in your meals. It is essential that you make a conscious effort to eliminate highly processed foods and eat healthy, chemical-free, fresh foods. This will allow you to get the most vitamins, minerals, and fiber content from the foods you eat and enjoy the greatest health benefits. If possible, I encourage you to buy organic, pesticide-free vegetables and fruits. Completely organic fruits and vegetables contain no chemicals to preserve their shelf life so they taste better and typically contain more nutrients. Did you know that the packaged lettuce, spinach, or cabbage you buy at the supermarket has been sprayed with preservatives?

Cattle that are grass-fed, like most of Argentina's beef, is much lower in fat content (about 20 percent lower) and tastes distinctively much better than most U.S. grain-fed beef. Did you know that much of our cattle, months prior to slaughter, are fed thousands of pounds of grain and have anabolic steroids implanted in their ear so they can gain around four hundred pounds and fetch a bigger profit? In recent years, E. coli contamination has risen due to the feed given to cattle, overcrowding of feedlots, poor sanitation in slaughterhouses, poorly trained workers, and reduced government regulation. The solution the USDA and meatpacking industry came up with is to start irradiating our beef with gamma rays. The poultry industry does not fare much better.

The point I'm trying to make is that you really need to take into consideration the source of your food. Our soils today are depleted due to overproduction, which means our fruits and vegetables have less vitamin and mineral content. I realize organic food is more expensive, but when considering the alternative, it might be worth it.

It is also very important to limit man-made,

processed foods. I'm referring to any food that comes in a can, wrapper, box, or bag. Processed foods tend to be high in fat, sodium, hydrogenated oil (trans fats), sugar, preservatives, and chemical flavorings.

Before World War II processed and fast foods had not yet proliferated and obesity was not an epidemic like it is today. By the end of the century, processed and fast-food sales dominated the $1 trillion food industry. To extend the shelf life of food and increase profits, food producers began adding fat, preservatives, and chemically-altered flavorings so we would crave these foods. In the fitness industry we call these foods empty calories because they are high in calories and bad fat and low on nutritional benefit.

Have you ever wondered why you could never eat just one Lay's potato chip? It has to do with the chemical flavoring. Chemists spend countless hours developing flavors and aromas that desensitize our taste buds and get us addicted to these foods. Our taste buds have a hard time telling our brain that they would rather have a piece of fruit or vegetables instead of Cap'n Crunch cereal, frozen pizza, or a convenience store hot dog.

Here are some examples of ideal menu choices along with the proper portions.

Seven Days of Menu Choices for You to Mix and Match

Zone Perfect 7-Day Meal Plan

DAY ONE
Breakfast
Scrambled egg whites (3–4)
Tomato (4 slices)
Grapefruit (½)

Morning Snack
Snack portion smoothie (½ cup of juice or 2% milk, scoop of whey protein)
Almonds (8–10)

Lunch
Mediterranean chicken breast (3 oz.)
Rice (¼ cup)
Vegetables (2 cups steamed)

Afternoon Snack
Tuna salsa salad (½ cup)
Medium apple

Dinner
Grilled ginger shrimp (4 oz.)
Broccoli (1 cup)
Red leaf, jicama, and carrot salad
Olive oil (1 tsp.)

DAY TWO
Breakfast
Plain 3 egg-white omelet with 1 oz. chicken or turkey sausage
One medium apple

Morning Snack
Applesauce (¼ cup)
Low-fat cheese (1 oz.)
Almonds (8–10)

Lunch
Chicken burrito with corn tortilla (3 oz. chicken with 1 tortilla)
Steamed vegetables (½ cup)

Afternoon Snack
Turkey meatballs (2 oz.) or turkey burger (2 oz.)
Blue corn chips (10)

Dinner
Roast turkey (3 oz.)
Sugar snap peas (½ cup)
Yellow squash (½ cup)
Romaine salad (1 cup)
Olive oil (1 tsp.)

DAY THREE
Breakfast
Wild berry smoothie (½ cup of juice or milk,
    scoop of whey protein)
Peanut butter (1½ tsp.)

Morning Snack
Hard-boiled egg
Grapes (½ cup)

Lunch
Chicken (3 oz.)
Steamed broccoli (2 cups)

Afternoon Snack
Tuna fish salad (2 oz.)
Baby carrots and celery (1 cup)

Dinner
Grilled salmon (4 oz.)
Sauteed vegetables (2 cups)
Fresh seasonal fruit salad (1 cup)

DAY FOUR
Breakfast
Cream of rice cereal (½ cup)
Chicken or turkey sausage (2 oz.)
Soy or 2% milk (4 oz.)

Morning Snack
Smoked salmon (1½ oz.)
Tomato slice (1)

Lunch
Chicken cacciatore (3 oz.)
Sliced tomatoes and cucumber (1½ cups)

Afternoon Snack
Hummus (½ cup)
Chicken (2 oz.)

Dinner
Grilled red snapper (4 oz.)
Vegetables (steamed or lightly sauteed, 1 cup)
Field green salad with olive oil (1 tsp.)

DAY FIVE
Breakfast
Scrambled eggs (½ cup)
Grilled ham (1 oz.)
Fresh seasonal fruit (1½ cups)

Morning Snack
Chicken or turkey slices (1 oz.)
Trail mix (¼ cup)

Lunch
Chicken salad (3 oz.)
Fruit of choice (1 piece or ½ cup chopped
    or sliced)

Afternoon Snack
Shrimp (3 oz.)
Lentils (½ cup)

Dinner
Turkey chili (4 oz.)
Mixed green salad (1 cup)

DAY SIX
Breakfast
Strawberry-banana smoothie (½ cup of juice or
    milk, scoop of whey protein)
Peanut butter (1½ tsp.)

Morning Snack

Peanut butter (1 tbsp.) with 3 celery stalks

Lunch

Garlic rosemary chicken (4 oz.)

Rice (¼ cup)

Vegetables (1 cup steamed or lightly sauteed)

Afternoon Snack

Blue corn chips (10)

Chicken salad (½ cup)

Dinner

Italian sausage and peppers (3 oz.; use chicken
   or turkey sausage)

Roasted tomato soup (1 cup)

Garden salad with cherry tomatoes (1 cup)

DAY SEVEN

Breakfast

Oatmeal (1 cup)

Soy or 2% Milk (½ cup)

Cottage cheese (½ cup)

Avocado (2 thin slices)

Morning Snack

Low-fat cheese (1 oz.)

1 medium apple

Lunch

Grilled garlic orange chicken (3 oz.)

Spinach africaine (1 cup)

Afternoon Snack

Edamame (1 cup in shells)

Dinner

Lemon basil turkey (4 oz.)

Steamed or lightly sauteed yellow
   squash/zucchini (1 cup)

Double pea soup (1 cup)

Supplements

Clients always ask me if they should be taking supplements. There are many theories about whether or not supplements are needed or if they even work. I do believe in supplementing your diet with just a few supplements, especially if you are under a lot of stress, for several reasons. Today we are busier than we've ever been and under greater stress, which depletes our body of vitamins. Also, our soils today are depleted of much of their vitamin and mineral content. Most of us buy our food from a supermarket or corner store. There is a large time lag between the time food is delivered from the farm to the store and then purchased by the consumer. In that time many fruits and vegetables lose a certain amount of their vitamin and mineral content, and on top of that many fruits and vegetables are picked early so they won't be overripe or spoil at the store, which also lessens vitamin and mineral content. That is why many fruits and vegetables, especially ones that spoil quickly, are sprayed with preservatives.

Keep in mind that you have to be careful of which types of supplements you purchase because many of them don't work effectively or contain exactly—or in the full amounts—what is on the label. It's all about the delivery system. Your body has a very difficult time assimilating and digesting hard chelated pills. Your digestive system can only digest approximately 60 percent of the solid pills. The rest go down the toilet, literally. So in order to not waste your money, I suggest purchasing capsules and time-released supplements whenever you can.

Herbs can also be beneficial when administered by a holistic doctor and when purchased from a reputable manufacturer. Remember, however, that just because herbs can be purchased over the counter doesn't mean they are innocuous and absolutely safe. Herbs can be just as powerful as drugs so they should be taken under the supervision of a physician or a holistic doctor.

Recommended Supplements for Women Per Day

Multivitamin (capsule): For many of you a multiple vitamin will suffice.

Vitamin C (capsule)	1,000 mg
B-12 (capsule)	250 mcg
B-1 (capsule)	100 mcg
B-6 (capsule)	100 mcg
Antioxidant (capsule)	250 mcg
Green Tea (capsule)	40 mg
Calcium (capsule)	1000 mg

Recommended Supplements for Men Per Day

Multivitamin (capsule): For many of you a multiple vitamin will suffice.

Vitamin C (capsule)	1,000 mg
B-12 (capsule)	250 mcg
B-1 (capsule)	100 mcg
B-6 (capsule)	100 mcg
Antioxidant (capsule)	250 mcg
Magnesium	200 mg

Ready, Set, Go!

These are the four principles of your Fat-Blasting Nutrition strategy. This is a way of eating that has a proven track record, is simple and realistic for a busy lifestyle, and supports rapid

---

THE FOUR PRINCIPLES

Principle 1:
Use the 40:30:30 ratio for each meal.

Principle 2:
Eat five small meals or snacks per day.

Principle 3:
Choose low glycemic carbohydrates over high glycemic carbohydrates.

Principle 4:
Choose fresh produce and lean meats.

---

fat loss and weight management. Now that you understand how much to eat, how often to eat, and in what proportion, let's align this way of eating with your goals. It is imperative that you have specific goals in mind. Remember, these goals need to be realistic, based on your lifestyle and body type. You need to visualize them and imagine what achieving them will look and feel like and how your life will be improved.

Your New Schedule

Let's start the planning process today. First, set a start date. How about tomorrow? I know you have not read the exercise chapters yet, but why not get a head start on your Fat-Blasting Nutrition program? Schedule your breakfast shortly after waking and then the remainder of your meals or snacks every 2½ to 3 hours. Remember, these meals are the key to your success. They are essential to creating the *you* that you are striving to become. When you look over your daily schedule, try to identify days or times that may be challenging for you. This will allow you to prepare something ahead of time so that you will have the food you need when you need it.

Overcoming Obstacles

You can overcome a lot of the obstacles you will face by proper planning. Part of my own planning involves spending a portion of my weekend preparing and cooking food for the upcoming week. If all I have to do is warm up my food, I am less likely to miss meals. I have found that if I prepare all of my proteins in advance, I can easily add a salad, cook some vegetables, or slice some fruit while I warm up my meal. In this way I always know that I can prepare a healthy, balanced meal in about ten to fifteen minutes.

Some other obstacles you may encounter could pertain to cravings or feeling unsatisfied by your meals. Since we are using the eyeball method for your meals and snacks, it may take a couple of weeks of experimentation to discover how much food you should eat at each meal.

Please trust this nutritional guideline and understand that you are retraining your body and your palate to adjust to a different way of eating. There will be an adjustment period before your cravings dissipate, but your taste buds will adjust and you will begin to thrive on not feeling overfull. If you are struggling with your nutrition strategy, go to www.bodyexpressmakeover .com for support and to get all your questions answered.

In review:

THE FOUR PRINCIPLES

Principle 1:
Use the 40:30:30 ratio for each meal.

Principle 2:
Eat five small meals or snacks per day.

Principle 3:
Choose low glycemic carbohydrates over high glycemic carbohydrates.

Principle 4:
Choose fresh produce and lean meats.

CHAPTER FIVE

SUPERFAST SCULPTING

Reducing body fat quickly can be accomplished only through increased cardiovascular activity. I think that by now we have all come to terms with the idea that dieting or strength training alone doesn't put us on the fast track for body-fat reduction. To burn excess body fat, an aerobic exercise component is required. My Superfast Sculpting System will show you how to reduce body fat fast and, in conjunction with the fat-blasting nutrition program, will help you attain your dream body. To expend stored fat, you must do some form of consistent aerobic exercise. The more aerobic exercise you do, the more fat you will burn.

This chapter will focus on the benefits of aerobic exercise and tell you what you need to do to reach your goals as fast as possible. Do you want to eliminate stress and regain a positive outlook on life? Do you want to improve your heart function dramatically? Do you want to feel revitalized and refreshed? If so, you must tap into your own power source. The quickest and most effective way to do so is through aerobic exercise.

When I say "aerobic exercise," I am not talking about a casual walk around the neighborhood, even though that too is beneficial. I am referring to any activity that elevates your heart rate, and gets your blood circulating for an extended period of time. From now on, I will refer to this activity as "cardio exercise."

What You Will Gain (and Lose) by Doing Cardiovascular Exercise

Cardio exercise has many benefits. Yes, it reduces body fat; but it also strengthens your heart muscle, reduces your stress level, helps you sleep better at night, and provides you with increased mental clarity. In just a few short weeks, you will notice considerable improvements in your health. You will achieve greater cardiovascular stamina and endurance, which means no more huffing and puffing when walking up a flight of stairs or playing with the kids. You will feel more energized throughout the day, your heart will become stronger, and your body will eliminate toxins more efficiently. You may also notice other benefits, such as a more positive outlook, greater tolerance, and having more patience to deal with daily stresses. And yes, you will probably be smiling more.

These results should be just as important to you as dropping body fat. After taking a brisk thirty-minute walk, you may not lose four inches from your waist; however, you will feel more energized and revitalized. That euphoric feeling is what will keep you exercising day after day, which will eventually result in you losing the excess body fat. Eventually, you might feel inspired to mix one-minute bursts of jogging into your walks. After a few days of this "burst training," you may feel so good that you incorporate three-minute intervals of running. After a few weeks of this kind of interval training, you may feel so energized and charged that you push yourself to even greater heights. In just a few weeks, you may be jogging for the entire thirty minutes, then forty-five minutes, and before you know it, you'll be running for an entire hour. Who knows, a 10K may follow! In a very short period of time, you will see that four-inch loss from your waistline.

The more you recognize and acknowledge the subtle changes in the way you feel and function on a day-to-day basis, the more motivated you will become to consistently do your cardiovascular exercise. This is a very important point that you really need to grasp and what may have been missing in any previous attempts to reduce body fat: results, no matter how small, are what will keep you motivated and empowered. Again, it is essential that you make some sort of notation in your journal after every exercise session, at least for the first six weeks. It does not have to be a novel. Just mention how you felt after each cardio session and what you noticed to be different in yourself.

The Mind/Body Connection

If you are just starting out on a cardiovascular conditioning regime, try to make observations about how your daily cardio sessions begin and end. As you begin each cardio session, you may find that it takes a few minutes to get going. Always begin slowly with a ten-minute warm-up to ease your body into the cardio activity and to allow your mind to follow. Everything your body does physically comes directly from your mind. Your brain tells your body how, when, and in what form it should move. Your mind also controls your emotional response to exercise, which is why the first ten minutes of every cardio session are crucial. It is in this period of time that you want to make sure your self-talk is positive. When I refer to self-talk, I am referring to the committee in your head that tells you how to respond emotionally to a physical challenge. Mentally, you may push yourself into starting the activity, but after only a few minutes, the torch will pass and your body will take over. As you look for greater fitness challenges, you may integrate intervals, the 100s, or the burst cardio, which we will talk about later in this chapter. A whole new perspective on mind/body cooperation will soon be revealed.

One thing I always tell my clients is that you need to approach each and every cardio exercise session with an open mind, without judging how it will go before you begin. Remember, be in the present, not in the future. Some days you will feel lethargic, distracted, or unmotivated and end up having an amazing cardio session because your body is raring to go. On other days, the opposite may be true: you may feel highly energized and end up having only a mediocre cardio session because your mind is alert but your body is fatigued. The bottom line is, all you have to do is show up and do the best you can on any given day. It's not about having the perfect workout; it's about doing the workout consistently. Trust me, you will always feel great after a cardio session if for no other reason than being proud of yourself for doing it despite not wanting to. So remember: no judgment and no expectations, just an open mind.

Many of us depend on outside sources to alter our mood. Whether through drugs or alcohol, prescription medication, the nicotine in tobacco, the caffeine in coffee, television, the Internet, video games, or the chemical compounds in the foods we eat, most of us rely on some stimulus to change our mental state. Cardiovascular exercise is more effective by far than any of the above-mentioned diversions in regard to altering your mental state positively. I believe that cardiovascular exercise is the healthiest mood-altering experience available. Take time to notice the internal shift that occurs after you do your cardiovascular exercise. If you do your cardio in the morning, you may find that you begin your day with a more positive attitude. It may encourage you to eat more healthfully throughout the day. If you do your cardio in the evening, more often than not you will find that the stress you encountered throughout the day will dissipate and obstacles won't feel as overwhelming as they did earlier in the day. Cardio exercise will soon become the one thing in your life that you cannot do without because your mind and body will crave it. I call this being "activated."

When I say "activated," I refer to feeling passionate about and engaged in life. It is when you feel the light has been turned on in your head and you have a passionate, confident, more positive outlook on life. This may happen only occasionally, or you may experience it every time you do your cardio exercise. You should also continue to feel activated for many

hours after your cardio session ends as your body will continue to burn extra calories even after you are through. If you take the time to notice this feeling of being activated, you will realize that it is happening more and more often.

You will also experience increased mental clarity and focus after doing your cardio sessions that will continue throughout the day. Have you ever had so much on your mind that you didn't know where to begin? Cardio exercise can help you organize your thoughts, think more creatively, and think "out of the box." As a result, you will feel more centered and at peace within yourself.

Your cardio sessions may be a little challenging at first, but I want you to push past your comfort level. If you exercise outdoors, you may have to overcome physical discomforts caused by weather and terrain. You may experience other physical obstacles, such as a low endurance level, shin splints, side aches, and the like. These are all initial obstacles that will subside in time. They may require you to make moment-to-moment adjustments and possibly alter your mode of cardio activity for a short period of time. These adjustments are precisely what keep you in the present moment.

This focus on the present, what is before you in the here and now, is a very powerful tool. By pushing yourself into a daily practice of being present, you may find yourself living more and more of your day in a positive state of mind. Being present is extremely important to avoiding injury when participating in any exercise activity. If you are distracted or not paying attention to the activity at hand, you are at risk of injuring yourself. When I am training my clients, I always make sure they are paying attention and engaged for the entire duration of their training session. Being present will also spill over into your personal, family, and business relationships.

Physical Results

I want you to periodically look at yourself in the mirror and take notice of even the smallest of physical changes. This is not the time to be critical. This is the time to praise yourself for the positive steps you are taking toward changing your body. You might feel that you are not losing fat in the right places or fast enough, but soon your fat loss will become more and more noticeable. I am confident that after only a short period of time, you will notice that your clothes are fitting a little more loosely. Within weeks, you may be wearing clothes that you couldn't fit into for years. In a few months, you may be shopping for a new wardrobe. That, by the way, is a very powerful and rewarding goal to have. Your goals do not have to be just physical, body-related goals; they can also be tangible ones that are by-products of losing body fat and altering your body's appearance.

Eliminating Fat

Superfast Sculpting is all about the process of reducing stored body fat through cardio exercise. It is the fastest, most efficient way to burn off the excess body fat that is covering the toned muscles you will develop through the Body Express strength training routines. There are many different philosophies about cardio exercise, and some physicians and experts say you don't need to do a significant amount of cardio to lose body fat. I disagree. After training clients for twenty years, I have discovered one very important truth: when clients consistently do their cardio exercise, they lose body fat quickly and are more likely to adhere to a healthy nutrition plan in the long term. When they don't consistently do cardio exercise, they don't lose body fat quickly and are much more likely to fail to reach their goal. This observation is based on my own experience as a personal trainer, nothing else.

It is imperative that you gradually work up to doing some form of cardiovascular activity four to six days per week. The Weekly Cardio Chart at the end of this chapter will help you determine how much cardio you will need to do based upon your goals, age, and fitness level. The Cooper Institute in Texas, a renowned fitness institution, claims studies have shown that the greatest protective benefits are found in at least thirty minutes of moderate to vigorous exercise daily. Recent studies have also shown that doing ten-minute bouts of cardio exercise several times throughout the day is just as effective as participating in just one session of cardio exercise per day. So break up your cardio sessions if you need to—just make sure you find a way to get in your allotted cardio exercise. Again, you do not have to run out and sign up for aerobics or spinning classes or purchase a treadmill unless that is what you want to do. All you have to do is get your body moving. Brisk walking is an excellent activity to get you started. Just increasing the number of steps you take per day is a great start.

Besides doing your allocated amount of cardio exercise, you need to look at other ways you can begin increasing your activity level. Look at what you do every day. Could you do more of the things you are already doing? If you play golf, could you walk the course instead of driving a cart? Could you use a shovel instead of a snowblower or a rake instead of a leaf blower? Would you like to or have you always wanted to do a certain sport or hobby? If you have always wanted to learn how to play tennis, for example, here is the perfect opportunity. Can you—or, more specifically, *will* you—do that?

The Body Express cardio and strength workouts are new activities that you will incorporate into your weekly schedule. In addition to your cardio sessions, is there something else you could do on your "off" days, perhaps a few times per week? Look at increasing your activity level as something you will do for the rest of your life. Make sure to choose activities that you enjoy. One of the primary reasons people stop participating in cardio exercise is that they force themselves to do activities they don't like, which is self-defeating behavior. Eventually, physical activity will become part of your daily routine. It is a commitment to yourself and your well-being.

Any added physical activity you perform will require your body to burn extra calories, and those calories should come from stored fat. So just get yourself moving—even if it is for a short, brisk walk. Take the dog for a long walk. Trust me, the dog won't complain. Schedule a lunch meeting six blocks away and walk to it. Hike on a nearby trail. Hop on that bicycle that's been sitting in your garage and ride around the neighborhood. Better yet, schedule a family bike ride. When was the last time you went bike-riding with your child or a friend? What about making your next vacation an active one that includes swimming, snorkeling, hiking, water sports, or a spa that has daily exercise classes? It's the little changes you make in your day-to-day life that will add up to huge benefits in the end. You will soon discover that when you make it a priority to be more active every day, it soon becomes a habit. Eventually, it becomes a lifestyle. You will begin making the time for new activities, and you will become attached to the way your more active lifestyle makes you feel.

Time Constraints

One of the biggest challenges I face with new clients is getting them to adhere to a consistent schedule of cardiovascular exercise, especially if they have been sedentary for a period of time. Of all the excuses I hear for not doing cardio exercise, not having enough time is by far the number-one excuse. Believe me, I understand that time is a very real obstacle. I have a very hectic schedule myself, but I always make the time to do sixty minutes of cardio, six days a week. I give myself one day a week of rest, and I suggest you do the same. I don't do cardio exercise to lose body fat. I do it to maintain my current weight, to reduce stress, and for all the other reasons listed earlier in the chapter.

It doesn't matter how crazy your day is; I promise that you either have the time or can make the time to do your cardio exercise if you really want to. I understand that most of us have a very busy, stressful lifestyle with career, family, and social obligations that require downtime; but you have to make cardio exercise a top priority if you want to become the *you* you've always dreamed of becoming. If you are still reading this book, I know you want to.

I want to tell you a true story. Recently, a

very dear friend of mine from college passed away from lupus erythematosus. For thirteen years she battled this disease with the courage of a warrior. She went through several surgeries, daily dialysis, and excruciating pain and never once complained about her suffering or her fate. She lost her battle a few days before having another surgery that might have saved her life. I might add that she had six root canals done at one time, a few days before her passing, without any anesthesia. That should give you an idea of the pain this woman endured during her fight with lupus. She was stricken with a disease, suffered immensely, and did everything in her power to live as long as possible. I might add that she had the most positive outlook on life of anyone I've ever met. She was not given a choice, but you *do* have a choice. You can choose to do everything in your power to live a long, healthy life. You can choose to try to be around long enough to watch your children grow up. I can't make you do this, but I can ask you to be honest with yourself when making the decision to consistently do your cardio exercise. Are the other priorities in your life more important than a long, healthy life?

I promise you can find the time, even if you are extremely busy. I recently was on the phone with a potential new client. She was fifty years old, sedentary, and needed to lose fifty pounds. She gave me every excuse in the book for why she couldn't start an exercise routine, and every excuse revolved around time and planning. I turned around and gave her every excuse why she should start an exercise program based upon—you guessed it—time and planning. She was so caught up in running her business that she didn't even realize that she had been seri-ously neglecting her health. She was a prime candidate for a heart attack, stroke, adult-onset type 2 diabetes, high blood pressure, and heart disease, just to name a few. She committed to finding one hour a day to devote to exercise, and she's stuck to it. Her health has improved, she feels great, and her business is still standing.

Do you spend a portion of your day winding down and relaxing? Perhaps you spend some time reading the morning paper while drinking coffee. Could you get your coffee to go on your way to the gym and read your paper on the bicycle? Perhaps you watch TV before or after you get home. Could you slip on a pair of headphones, take a brisk walk, and listen to the evening news or sports report on the radio? Could you occasionally replace your cocktail hour with an evening jog with your spouse? Could you wake up a little earlier and get in your cardio before work? Could you play a game of tennis with a business associate rather than sitting across a restaurant table from him or her in a meeting? Sometimes it takes a little creativity, but I assure you, there *is* time in your day.

If time is of concern (and it is for everyone), take another look at the caloric expenditure of your exercise. If you walk one mile, you will expend approximately 100 calories. If you run the same mile, you might expend 105 or even 110 calories. In terms of the caloric expenditure, it is not much of a difference. However, in terms of the time it takes to expend those calories, the difference is far greater. Depending on your pace, it might take fifteen to thirty minutes to walk that mile. If you were jogging, you could burn off those same calories in around ten minutes. Burning off calories in the fastest possible time is the entire premise of the Body Express

Makeover. Superfast Sculpting involves restructuring your daily cardiovascular activity to expend the maximum number of calories in the least amount of time.

Likes and Dislikes

The second most popular excuse for not doing cardio exercise is that people just don't like it. I understand that sweating and pushing yourself physically might not be first on your list of fun activities. However, if you participate in activities that you enjoy rather than ones that you don't, you will be more apt to adhere to a consistent cardio routine. If you hate being indoors, take your cardio outdoors. There are numerous activities that can be done outside, such as walking, jogging, biking, hiking, and Rollerblading. If you absolutely hate jogging, you can participate in group exercise classes, such as spinning, kickboxing, or a dance class. You can learn a new skill such as martial arts, boxing, or belly dancing. How about purchasing one of the hundreds of exercise videos that you can follow at home? It is vitally important that you participate in cardio exercise that you enjoy, or you will most certainly find a reason not to do it.

If you can't seem to find any activity that interests you, you need to take a look at your relationship to cardio activity. Be honest with yourself. What is it you hate about doing cardio exercise? What can you do to change your attitude about it? Write down how you feel about it in your journal, and see what truths surface. It may be that you disliked phys ed in elementary school and have carried that feeling into your adult life. Maybe you had a bad experience playing a sport and decided that you would never

again participate in any sports. Maybe the last time you started an exercise regimen, you didn't see results fast enough. The truth is that most likely you will find that your attitude toward cardio activity has been affected in one way or another by some previous event or situation. It is important to remember that whatever transpired in the past does not have to determine the present. Today you are embarking on the Body Express Makeover training system with a renewed sense of confidence and a strong commitment to succeed. You can do it. You do have the heart and the will to succeed.

Another issue that stands in the way of consistent cardiovascular exercise is boredom. Many of my clients cite boredom as one of the top reasons for not doing their cardio activity. However, there is a way to make your cardio exercise more interesting. For instance, do a mode of cardio that allows you to read your favorite novel or magazine. My favorite is the StepMill. Since my days are so busy, I don't get much time to just sit, relax, and read a book. Most of my reading is done in the sixty minutes on the Step-Mill. If you were to set a goal to read a book every couple of weeks or study a new language, wouldn't that make the time fly by? What about listening to books on tape? Most large bookstores have an entire section devoted to books on tape.

I have also found that music is one of the best motivators when it comes to doing cardio exercise consistently. Wear headphones, and listen to your favorite music. Change the music often so that you don't get into a pattern where your cardio becomes boring. Your experience will always be different since music evokes an emotional response from us. Get creative and find what works best for you. The biggest pitfall is to get lazy and listen to the same radio station or the same three CDs over and over again. There are ways to combat boredom; you just have to be willing to do them.

Another important factor in eliminating boredom is to cross train. I am a big proponent of cardio cross training, which really just means frequently changing your mode of cardio activity. Doing the same activity over and over again can become mindless, which leads to boredom. Cross training is a fun and exciting way not only to liven up your workouts but to learn new and challenging skills, reduce the risk of overuse injuries, and help maintain a consistent cardio routine. This might mean doing fifteen minutes on three to four different machines in one cardio session or changing your mode of doing cardio every couple of days. It might mean mixing jumping rope with aerobics classes or hiking with swimming. The nice thing about cross training is that you make the choice as to what activities you would like to cross train in and for how long you'd like to participate in them.

Cross training is also important in preventing overuse injuries. As you embark on a new program of cardio exercise, especially if you have not been very active for a while, you may experience minor aches and pains. The body is very much like a machine: repetitive use of muscles with the same activity and the same amount of resistance at the same speed wears down joints and strains the muscles where the greatest amount of stress is located. When you cross train, as opposed to doing the same activity over and over, you have a better chance of avoiding overuse syndrome of any one particular muscle group.

A physical activity that can often result in overuse injuries is running. One example is shin splints. Some people who use running as their primary mode of physical activity can develop shin splints. These are caused by minuscule tears in the muscle, which cause pain in the shins that can extend from the ankle all the way up to the knee. Another injury is runner's knee, which is a sharp pain located directly under or surrounding the patella (kneecap). This pain is typically the result of inflammation of muscle tissue due to overuse and overpronation. Both of these injuries can become chronic or develop into something worse if not addressed. The musculoskeletal system needs time to recuperate from the mechanical stresses of running. One way to avoid them is to refrain from running every day and work some other mode of cardio exercise into your routine. Over the years, I have learned to use cross training as a way of preventing injuries. By participating in a variety of activities, I decrease downtime due to injury and pain. If you do run, make sure you have good running shoes that are right for your particular stride and foot placement. You also want to replace your shoes frequently because they break down. A good rule of thumb is to buy new shoes every four to six months, depending on how many miles per week you run.

We have all experienced that plateau where we just can't seem to make any significant changes in our bodies. This is especially noticeable if you are trying to lose just a few extra pounds. Varying your cardio activities can be one of the solutions. When an activity becomes routine, we tend to slack off or not push as hard, which in turn limits our progress. It is necessary to gradually and consistently push your body to work a little harder. Over time your body will become stronger, and you will have greater stamina.

By participating in different modes of cardio activities, you will be more enthusiastic and eager to do them, and your cardio workouts will become much more enjoyable. This is important in this day and age, where everything needs to be done yesterday. If you hit that plateau, don't get frustrated. Try a different cardio activity and break through the barrier. Eventually you will find several cardio activities you enjoy.

How Can I Burn the Most Calories in the Shortest Time?

Cardiovascular exercise has two distinct categories: *aerobic* exercise and *anaerobic* exercise. Both of these terms refer to, and are directly related to, the frequency at which your heart is beating. Aerobic exercise (with oxygen) is your long-term energy source and requires the utilization of oxygen. The term *anaerobic* (without oxygen) is your short-term energy source due to oxygen debt. The molecule ATP is your primary energy source. Due to the lack of oxygen, your body can only sustain this high level of cardiovascular output for a brief period of time.

A perfect example of these two categories of exercise is best illustrated in the 400-yard dash or a two-to-three minute maximal-effort sprint. Approximately 50 percent of the energy comes from aerobic sources and 50 percent from anaerobic sources. However, in a ten-minute maximal-effort activity, the anaerobic component drops to only 15 percent due to lack of oxygen. Basically what this demonstrates is that with aerobic training the muscles become more

efficient in burning fat, and fatigue is slower because glycogen and oxygen are not used as quickly during exercise.

The reason for defining these two forms of exercise is so you understand that most of your cardiovascular exercise will be done in an aerobic state. However, going into and out of the anaerobic state will help increase your cardiovascular stamina and endurance, thus strengthening your heart and raising your overall fitness level. In essence, you want to do aerobic exercise that is just out of your comfort zone and every once in a while push yourself even further for short spurts. This type of cardiovascular training allows you to do what I call "raising the bar": you need to continually strive to push yourself past your self-imposed limitations to achieve your weight loss goals, make consistent progress, and stay motivated to exercise regularly.

The level at which your body burns calories most efficiently will vary, as will how long you can sustain that level, depending upon your gender, age, and fitness condition. The cardiovascular and respiratory systems work together to transport oxygen throughout the body. This process is called oxygen uptake or consumption. Oxygen consumption is called VO_2. Maximal oxygen consumption (VO_2 max) is the best way to gauge cardiovascular fitness. It is the highest rate of oxygen transport at a person's maximal physical exertion. Someone who is not very fit may be able to sustain an intensity level of only 40 percent of VO_2 max, whereas someone who is in mediocre shape may be able to sustain 60 percent of VO_2 max and a very fit person may sustain 80 percent of VO_2 max. Therefore, the best intensity level for you is the level that you can sustain for an extended period of time that challenges you throughout most of the entire cardio session. The key is to raise that intensity level gradually and continually, thus forcing you and your body to work harder.

There is an equation that determines what your maximum heart rate should be. I will walk you through this equation so that you can determine where your most efficient levels are. You may want a calculator to help determine these numbers. I also suggest that you write these numbers in your journal so that you can refer back to them later and keep track of the changes in your heart rate levels. At most, the human heart can beat only 220 times per minute. Each year you are alive, your maximum heart rate gets lower and lower. To determine what your maximum heart rate should be, simply subtract your age from 220. For instance, if you are 40 years old, your maximum heart rate would be 180 ($220 - 40 = 180$). To achieve maximum fat-burning efficiency, you should work toward keeping your heart rate around 75 percent of your VO_2 max for the majority of your cardio session. Let's determine what that means in terms of your personal target range. Using the example of a person who is 40 years of age, multiply the heart rate of 180 by .75. The ideal aerobic level for a 40-year-old would thus be about 135 heartbeats per minute. It may take a while to get to that level, but don't get discouraged. You are still burning calories, even if you are working at a lower level.

When your heart rate nears 80 to 85 percent of your maximum, you begin to move into the anaerobic state. When you reach this threshold, you can sustain it for only a brief period of time. Throughout your cardio sessions, you will primarily be in your aerobic zone. However, don't get worried about going into and out of your anaerobic zone at times, because by doing so you will increase your level of cardiovascular stamina and endurance, strengthening your heart muscle while still burning calories.

Monitoring Your Heart Rate

Now that you have calculated your ideal heart rate range, you need to know how to find your pulse. There are three methods of determining how many times per minute your heart is beating. Two of these methods can be done manually with the aid of a clock or stopwatch; the third utilizes a small machine. You can take your own pulse at two points on the body: at the wrist and on the neck. Finding the right spots takes a little practice, but after you have identified them and become familiar with them, they will prove to be fairly easy indicators of your heart rate. The point on the wrist is sometimes easier to find. Find the point at which your forearm meets the hand. Place your first and middle fingers in the middle of that area. (Never use your thumb, as it has its own pulse.) You will feel a tendon or even several tendons in your wrist. Move your fingers slowly to the inside portion of your wrist until you can find the pulse at its strongest point.

The other point at which you can accurately measure your pulse is in the neck, at the carotid artery. I actually find it easier to take the pulse here. To find this artery, locate the point where the front of your neck muscles meets your throat. Move your fingers slowly up the inside neck muscle until you find the point at which the pulse is the strongest. With your finger on either of these two spots, refer to a clock with a second hand or to a stopwatch. Count the number of your heartbeats for fifteen seconds. Then multiply that number by four to determine your heart rate per minute. A third option is to use a heart monitor. There are a number of heart monitors on the market. I personally like using these devices, as opposed to taking my own pulse, because they are typically very accurate and easy to use. The one I use is part of my wristwatch. All I have to do is look at my wristwatch, and I can see my heart rate instantly.

How Long Should I Exercise?

My recommendation is to follow the cardiovascular activity chart at the end of this chapter. This chart takes into account your primary goal, age, and current fitness level. The cardio chart is to be used as a basic guideline. You can always do more than is outlined in the chart, but make a concerted effort not to do less if you want to see fast results. The cardio chart is divided into categories based upon your fitness condition, from sedentary to extreme athlete. I suggest spending a maximum of six weeks in each category and then moving up to the next category until you reach maintenance level. The key is to really push through each category as quickly as possible. Remember, challenging yourself and raising the bar are essential to realizing your goals and especially to losing body fat. You do not need to reach the advanced or extreme category to attain your goals. All you need to do is move up to a category that is challenging but sustainable. As a matter of fact, most of you will attain amazing results just by moving up to the intermediate level.

I don't recommend more than one hour of cardio exercise per day unless you are an athlete or are performing extra aerobic activity to prepare for a social event or fitness competition. It's especially important to take baby steps if you are just embarking on an exercise regimen. If you have been exercising steadily for a while, use your own judgment, based on the cardiovascular chart and common sense. If you push too hard and too fast, you will risk burning yourself out, which is counterproductive. Understand that the body needs time for recovery and rest to be able to operate efficiently. Also, always make sure to do ten minutes of warm-up and cool-down activity.

Superfast Sculpting

With Superfast Sculpting, you will burn calories quickly and improve your heart health in the process. If you are just beginning, I suggest simply walking at first. Every once in a while, work yourself up into a light jog or maybe even a short run, and really get your heart rate up for ten to sixty seconds or until you feel you just can't keep up the pace anymore. Every few days, add one more short spurt. Remember, this is a process. As your cardiovascular stamina increases, the 2-in-1 exercise routines will also become easier to complete.

Interval Training

Now let's talk about how to spice up your cardio workouts and make them more effective and challenging. Interval training is extremely beneficial. It doesn't matter if you are walking, jogging, rowing, or biking. Simply change the pace of your movement every one to three minutes. Start slowly and warm up your body. Make your effort strenuous for one to three minutes, in the 70 to 80 percent VO_2 max range, then slow down to the level at which you normally do your cardio workout. Intersperse shorter periods when you are in an anaerobic state, 80 percent to 85 percent of your VO_2 max, for thirty to sixty seconds. If you happen to be using gym equipment for your cardiovascular exercise, most have an interval program option. Some machines' monitors simulate going up and down hills with an incline function. If you are on a treadmill, climber, stationary bike, or elliptical trainer, the program will increase and decrease the incline or resistance on its own. Raising the incline is also a great way to raise your heart rate and do interval training. As your cardiovascular stamina and endurance increase, you will also want to gradually increase the duration of your cardio sessions. When you have achieved a fitness level that allows you to do interval training for a sustained period of time, you will be ready for a greater challenge.

100s Training

The 100s workout is a unique, challenging way to get your cardiovascular and strength training in at the same time. I created this program to save time for my celebrity clients who need to get fit fast. You can easily do the 100s while walking outdoors or on a treadmill. However, on a treadmill be very careful to walk at a pace in which you can maintain balance easily. Begin walking at a slower than normal pace that is challenging yet allows you to keep your balance. Typically, on a treadmill this speed will be between 2 and 3 mph. You can also add an incline, which targets the lower body a little more, but make sure to adjust the speed so that you can still maintain your balance. Be careful when doing 100s for the first time. Walk at a slower pace, and use extremely light hand weights (dumbbells) because you will partake in strength-training activity.

Many of you will not be able to complete 100 repetitions of each exercise at first. That is the ultimate goal. I want you to have something to work up to so you continually challenge yourself. Start by doing only 25 repetitions of each exercise. When you master 25 repetitions, add increments of 10 to 20 repetitions every few times you do 100s. If you are an extreme exerciser, try this on a stationary bike or stair climber or just walking upstairs. You can utilize hand weights, water bottles, or even soup cans if necessary. The following is the sequence of strength training exercises you will engage in while performing whatever cardio exercise you have chosen (treadmill, stationary bike, or stair walking):

Shoulder Presses	100 repetitions
Biceps Curls	100 repetitions
Side Lateral Raises	100 repetitions
Triceps Extensions	100 repetitions
Front Lateral Raises	100 repetitions
Double Triceps Kickbacks	100 repetitions
Rear Lateral Raises	100 repetitions

After you are through with the above routine, stop walking and perform the following:

Squats with Calf Raises	100 repetitions
Crunches	100 repetitions
Push-ups	To failure

Immediately slow your pace and cool down for three to five minutes. Afterward, be sure to stretch all muscle groups worked during this program with one of the flexibility programs in chapter 11.

> The 100s program is equivalent in caloric expenditure to a 1½-hour jog. Depending on your intensity level and the number of repetitions you perform, you can expend anywhere from 500 to 1,000 calories in about thirty to sixty minutes.

Burst Cardio

Burst Cardio is unique and challenging because you integrate extremely high-intensity cardiovascular activity with highly demanding strength training. I recommend Burst Cardio only if your fitness level is advanced or extreme. Use light weights, start with 25 repetitions of each exercise, and work your way up in increments.

Start with three minutes of any high-intensity activity. When I say "high-intensity," I mean any activity that elevates your heart rate beyond your normal capacity into a range that you can sustain for only three to five minutes at best (80 to 90 percent of your maximum heart rate). This might be jumping rope, sprints, running stairs, hitting a heavy bag, or box jumps (plyometrics) to name a few. After three minutes, do:

Shoulder Presses	100 repetitions
Biceps Curls	100 repetitions

Do three more minutes of high-intensity cardiovascular activity, then do:

Side Lateral Raises	100 repetitions
Triceps Extensions	100 repetitions

Do three more minutes of high-intensity cardiovascular activity, then do:

Front Lateral Raises	100 repetitions
Double Triceps Kickbacks	100 repetitions

Do three more minutes of high-intensity cardiovascular activity, then do:

Rear Lateral Raises	100 repetitions
Squats with Calf Raises	100 repetitions

Do three more minutes of high-intensity cardiovascular activity, then do:

Crunches	100 repetitions
Push-ups	To failure

Immediately slow your pace and cool down for three to five minutes. Then stretch utilizing one of the stretching programs in chapter 11.

> Burst Cardio is equivalent in caloric expenditure to sprinting fifteen 200-yard dashes. Depending on your intensity level and the number of repetitions performed, you will expend anywhere from 600 to 1,200 calories in about forty to sixty minutes.

Ready, Set, Go!

Now you understand why you must get more physically active and partake in cardio exercise consistently. The form of exercise can be as simple as a brisk walk or as strenuous as Burst Cardio or the 100s. Open your calendar and look at your schedule for tomorrow. Find twenty to thirty minutes to do your cardio exercise. Just schedule it into your day; block out the time and mark it in your calendar. By scheduling it, you become accountable to yourself.

Schedule blocks of time for your cardio sessions for the remainder of this week. When you sit down with your calendar this weekend and plan your upcoming week, be certain to schedule in your cardio sessions. Make this commitment to yourself; make yourself accountable by scheduling in the time. This is exactly what I do week after week: I schedule my cardio and strength training workouts every single day.

Your New Schedule

You will need to do some planning and scheduling. That is why your calendar is of supreme importance. Again, on the weekend, block out an hour or so to make a plan for the upcoming week. Schedule all of your cardio sessions and all your meals or snacks. Take note if any exercise sessions conflict with any appointments, meetings, or events you have planned and adjust accordingly. You may need to stock the refrigerator at work, take your own lunch to work, or keep meal replacement bars in your desk or briefcase or in the glove compartment of your car.

It is essential that you eat every 2½ to 3 hours. In the next chapter, we will talk about strength training and my revolutionary 2-in-1 exercise routines.

WEEKLY CARDIO CHART

	Sedentary	Beginning	Intermediate	Advanced	Extreme
Ages 20–30:					
Lose body fat	20 minutes x 3 days	30 minutes x 4 days	40 minutes x 5 days	50 minutes x 6 days	60 minutes x 6 days
Sculpt and tone	20 minutes x 3 days	30 minutes x 3 days	40 minutes x 4 days	40 minutes x 5 days	40 minutes x 6 days
Build muscle	20 minutes x 3 days	20 minutes x 3 days	30 minutes x 3 days	30 minutes x 3 days	30 minutes x 4 days
Improve heart health	20 minutes x 3 days	20 minutes x 3 days	30 minutes x 3 days	30 minutes x 4 days	30 minutes x 5 days
Ages 30–40:					
Lose body fat	20 minutes x 3 days	30 minutes x 3 days	40 minutes x 4 days	45 minutes x 5 days	45 minutes x 6 days
Sculpt and tone	20 minutes x 3 days	25 minutes x 3 days	30 minutes x 4 days	35 minutes x 5 days	35 minutes x 6 days
Build muscle	20 minutes x 3 days	20 minutes x 3 days	30 minutes x 3 days	30 minutes x 4 days	30 minutes x 4 days
Improve heart health	20 minutes x 3 days	20 minutes x 3 days	20 minutes x 4 days	25 minutes x 4 days	30 minutes x 5 days
Ages 40–50:					
Lose body fat	20 minutes x 3 days	25 minutes x 3 days	30 minutes x 4 days	35 minutes x 5 days	45 minutes x 5 days
Sculpt and tone	20 minutes x 3 days	25 minutes x 3 days	25 minutes x 4 days	30 minutes x 5 days	30 minutes x 5 days
Build muscle	20 minutes x 3 days	20 minutes x 3 days	20 minutes x 4 days	30 minutes x 4 days	30 minutes x 4 days
Improve heart health	20 minutes x 3 days	20 minutes x 3 days	25 minutes x 4 days	25 minutes x 4 days	30 minutes x 5 days
Ages 50+:					
Lose body fat	20 minutes x 3 days	20 minutes x 4 days	25 minutes x 4 days	30 minutes x 4 days	40 minutes x 5 days
Sculpt and tone	20 minutes x 3 days	25 minutes x 3 days	25 minutes x 4 days	30 minutes x 5 days	30 minutes x 5 days
Build muscle	20 minutes x 3 days	20 minutes x 3 days	20 minutes x 4 days	20 minutes x 4 days	30 minutes x 4 days
Improve heart health	20 minutes x 3 days	20 minutes x 3 days	20 minutes x 4 days	20 minutes x 4 days	30 minutes x 5 days

CHAPTER SIX

2-IN-1 TONING

The Body Express Makeover is all about time. The strength training programs are uniquely designed to save you time. By far the most revolutionary aspect of the Body Express Makeover is the unique 2-in-1 total body workouts. I have created three programs for both men and women that will burn

fat while toning and sculpting every muscle in your body. Every exercise in my unique 2-in-1 Strength Training system is a multimuscle group exercise that provides you with a highly effective and efficient workout in the shortest time possible. This revolutionary system works two or more muscle groups simultaneously, so that you can do a complete total-body workout in as little as ten minutes.

If you have ever worked out in a gym setting or with a personal trainer, you know what a time-consuming process it can be. Traditionally, strength training exercises use free weights or weight-bearing machines. Usually, you go from one machine to the next and work one muscle or muscle group at a time. You then move on to another machine to work a different muscle group. Normally you do this in some sort of order, spending several minutes on each exercise, resting in between sets.

With the 2-in-1 program, you will be working two or more opposing body parts simultaneously. For example, in one exercise you will work your biceps, quadriceps, hamstrings, and glutes all at the same time with two movements.

In another exercise you will work your abs and chest together. In short, throughout the entire workout you will be multitasking. To make this an exciting, fun, and challenging exercise system, I mixed in yoga postures with martial arts stances and kicks, strength training exercises with aerobic intensity and Pilates techniques with core training. The result is an extremely effective strength training routine that will help you attain your goals faster than you could ever imagine. It is an entirely unique and revolutionary discipline that blends Eastern and Western philosophies with stamina and agility.

The Toning Revolution

The 2-in-1 exercises are a revolution in fitness. They dispel many commonly held beliefs about focus, challenge preconceptions about form, and obliterate the traditional model of exercise. So whether you have been sedentary, exercise regularly, or are an expert in the field, my unique 2-in-1 exercises will challenge you to excel and achieve amazing results.

It doesn't matter if you are just beginning

an exercise regime or if you are an extreme fitness fanatic, you will be challenged by these strength routines. At whatever fitness level you begin, you will push beyond your comfort zone, beyond training plateaus, and, more important, beyond whatever goals you may have previously set for yourself. The 2-in-1 Body Express routine is simply the most exciting, revolutionary, time-efficient, and effective exercise system to date.

The Beauty of Strength Training

With a foundation built upon Fat-Blasting Nutrition, Superfast Sculpting, and now the 2-in-1 Strength Training exercises, there is no goal that is out of your reach. It is essential to put another piece of your transformation puzzle firmly in place. Strength training utilizes resistance to build lean muscle mass. It is not optional but rather an essential component of your lifestyle transformation.

Strength training will strengthen and tone every muscle in your body, while your nutrition and cardiovascular programs will help reduce body fat. Everyone can have a set of well-defined triceps, calves, and chest muscles. As you eliminate more and more fat, the shape and tone of the muscles underneath will come to the surface. Strength training will tone, shape, and sculpt your muscles so that by the time you (and everyone else) can see them, they will look great. Don't worry; you will not build "bulk"—unless of course that is your goal. You will create beautiful, elongated muscles. This is done through the addition of muscle density, not necessarily by building larger muscles. By increasing your

muscle density, you will become stronger, more defined, and more toned, and your muscles will have a more attractive, symmetrical shape.

Muscle density (lean muscle mass) has no relationship to muscular bulk, so have no fear that this strength program will make you look like a bodybuilder. You can, however, bulk up if that is your goal just by increasing the weight and the number of times you utilize the 2-in-1 exercises every week. Every muscle in your body will become denser without growing in size. The muscles in your body are made up of thousands of strands of muscle fibers. Like the woven fibers that make up a rope, the individual fibers can be fragile, like yarn, or have density and strength similar to bundled wire. When you lift weights or use resistance, it causes rips and tears in the muscles on a microscopic level. When these minuscule tears heal, a denser, stronger muscle fiber is created.

Strength training is truly the only way to dramatically increase muscle density and, in doing so, create greater definition, tone, and shape. In addition to helping you look great, strength training provides you with many other benefits.

The Infinite Benefits of Strength Training

My exercise system will create lean muscle mass. This lean muscle mass will act as a furnace to burn body fat. By adding a pound of lean muscle mass, you will also be lowering your percentage of body fat. The more lean muscle mass you gain, the more your percentage of body fat will be reduced.

These exercises were designed to increase your metabolism, or metabolic rate, in two ways. First, you will create more lean muscle. Second, the way in which your body synthesizes protein will be completely transformed. Your metabolic rate is one of several important factors that determine your weight. It refers to the rate at which your body burns calories or utilizes energy. Lean muscle requires the consumption of many more calories than body fat, and as your lean muscle mass increases, you will naturally burn off more calories—even while you are sleeping. Up to thirty-six hours after you work out, you will still be burning over 20 percent more calories than normal.

A 2003 Finnish study found that protein synthesis (the process that creates muscular density) increases by more than 21 percent three hours after a workout, while protein breakdown increases by 17 percent. The combination is called "protein turnover," and it uses up a great deal of energy (calories). The short but intense 2-in-1 exercises are precisely the kind of workout that creates a faster metabolism.

In addition to creating lean muscle mass, the 2-in-1 Body Express routines deliver many other health-related benefits. They will increase your bone density and eliminate or offset the risk of osteoporosis. During these short but intense workouts, you will place greater impact on your joints and tendons. This is not the kind of impact that causes injury but rather the type of impact that creates greater bone density, strengthens joints, and reinforces your tendons. These 2-in-1 exercise routines will also cause an increase in the amount of antioxidants (naturally occurring disease fighters) in your blood-stream and will consequently boost your immune system.

The 2-in-1 Body Express Workout

The 2-in-1 exercise routines I have created eliminate the notion that only one muscle group can be worked at any one time. This revolutionary system works many muscle groups simultaneously, so that you can get a total body workout in minutes rather than hours. By performing these exercises back to back, with very little rest, you will increase your heart rate and expend more calories. The result is a powerful blend of disciplines that strengthens, tones, and sculpts your muscles—and does so in the most time-efficient manner ever devised.

These programs do not require that you join a gym or do them in any type of public setting. They can be performed in the privacy of your own home or behind the closed door of your office or hotel room. Since you will be using opposing limbs and multiple body parts, they may feel slightly awkward at first. I want you to expect this and not get discouraged. This training system is like nothing you've ever done before, and there will be a learning curve. Each time you perform one of these routines, you will become more proficient. After just a few times, your form will improve and you will begin to feel comfortable with each routine. Before you know it, you will be able to perform these exercises with grace and finesse.

10/20/30

There are three routines that are designed to last ten, twenty, or thirty minutes. Whoever told you that you need an hour in the gym to get a full workout? By splitting your focus and performing several different exercises at once, you can get a total body workout in just ten minutes.

Each 10, 20, and 30 2-in-1 Routine has twenty exercises—ten for women, and ten for men. I developed two different sets because one generally does not train the female body in the same way as the male body. Women are typically more concerned with their hips, thighs, buttocks, triceps, and lower abdominals, whereas men are usually more concerned with their chest, arms, and entire abdominal region. For the first six weeks of the Total Body Express Makeover program, stick with your gender-specific exercises in the exact order they are presented here. Once you are very familiar with each gender-specific exercise and routine, you can try the opposite gender's exercises if they target an area of the body you feel you need to focus on. Many of the exercises are interchangeable between genders. In the next chapter I will discuss how you can customize and modify many of the 2-in-1 strength exercises.

The 10 Routine

Like all three routines, the 10 Routine provides you with a series of ten different exercises to be done in ten minutes. All of these exercise routines were designed to warm you up with the first exercise of each routine, then strengthen and tone every muscle group in a specially designed order.

This entry-level routine is your introduction to the Body Express exercises. At the beginning, if in doubt, use the Weekly Exercise Chart at the end of this chapter to determine how many 10 Routines you should do each week. The Weekly Exercise Chart is a guide to the minimum amount of resistance training you should do, based upon your age and present fitness condition. By no means should you feel as though you have to follow the chart exactly. I would prefer that you customize the exercise routines to meet your goals, which I will help you to do in the next chapter. You will find yourself relying on the 10 Routine on days when your time is very limited. The 10 Routine can easily be performed at home, in your hotel room, or even in your office as the perfect ten-minute break to recharge your energy level.

The 20 Routine

The 20 Routine is a little more challenging than the 10 Routine. As you first begin integrating the 20 Routine into your exercise regime, it will probably push you past your comfort zone. After only a few times, you will notice a dramatic increase in your strength, stamina, and overall performance of the routine itself. While it may be difficult the first few times, soon this twenty-minute session should become your workout of choice.

Unlike the 10 Routine, which is really designed to be an entry-level routine, or performed when your time is extremely limited, the 20 Routine is designed to be a more strenuous exercise session and is highly effective for toning and sculpting each and every muscle group. If you really want to sculpt your body and lose both fat and inches, the 20 Routine is the primary routine to follow due to its time efficiency and overall muscle group training. If you want to build muscle mass, all you have to do is increase the amount of weight you use and the number of times you do the 20 Routine every week.

The 30 Routine

The 30 Routine is more challenging than the 20 Routine and was designed to be utilized after the 20 Routine is mastered. For those who seek the ultimate challenge, this thirty-minute routine can be made even more difficult by doing the exercises back to back with little or no rest. It will take time to reach the level of strength and endurance required to complete the 30 Routine but eventually you will master it and feel empowered beyond your expectations.

The Transformation Workshop

In training you to become your own coach, part of my job is to help you transform much more than your appearance. I suggest that when doing the 10, 20, or 30 Routine, you use your journal to make observations about what you experienced during your workout. Did you get winded? Did a certain muscle group give out before others? Is one side of your body stronger than the other? Could you finish the routine? How did you feel afterward? Writing these observations down in your journal will help you to understand your body better and assist you to determine which exercises require you to be a little more attentive. Using the same milestones suggested in previous chapters, I contend that the 10, 20, and 30 Routines are a very rapid and effective means of transforming your body and your life. The 2-in-1 training system will overhaul your emotional, intellectual, and spiritual life. Let me explain.

Power Tools

You need to be hyperaware of any subtle or unsubtle changes and improvements in the connection between mind and body. In your journal, I want you to note any shift toward a more positive outlook on life. Be aware of how your stress level decreases. Assess your energy levels and note new feelings of vitality. Become more aware of your increased mental clarity. Last, see if you have more balance in your life. Do you still feel scattered, as if you are being pulled in several different directions at once, or do you feel a certain calm in the air?

The 2-in-1 Body Express routines were designed to target these areas of your life and to help you develop these power tools. Eventually, I don't want you to simply go through an exercise routine, I want you to be present and aware of what your body is doing so that you will develop a closer working relationship and connection between your mental and physical functions.

The Mind/Body Connection

In the beginning, exercising may be awkward because you will be trying to follow the directions while looking at pictures of each exercise. This is a great example of our normal body/mind connection. It is one in which our cerebral approach forces the body to move against its will. Our bodies are naturally subservient to the commands of the mind. Everything starts with the mind passing down signals to your body to perform some physical task.

Imagine you wanted to learn how to dance and signed up for classes. In your first class, you might be forced to study painted footsteps on the floor. You would first clod your way through—one, two, three, four—with all the grace of Frankenstein's monster. Soon your body would begin to interpret and assimilate the music on its own. As your body learned the steps, you would realize that the more you think about what you're doing, the less fluid it becomes. You would eventually learn to stop trying to force your body to perform and simply let it do what it's been trained to do. And presto, you'd be dancing—really dancing! As you continue to practice, you stop thinking about what you're doing and just do it. You will go through a similar journey with the Body Express 2-in-1 exercises. You will come to a place where your body eventually leads the way. When you reach this point, your mind is no longer an observer but an active and equal participant.

Shift

In a literal sense, you will be constantly shifting your body as you perform these routines. You will shift your weight, your stance, and your position. You will shift your intention as you go from one exercise to another. In each exercise you will shift to a completely different set of muscle groups. This constant shifting will develop greater mental and physical agility.

The first shift may be your inner voice, changing its tune from "I can't do this" to "I'm really getting this." You will feel a greater sense of accomplishment. My hope is that it will extend past your exercise sessions and into your daily life. You may find yourself coming up with creative alternatives to overcome obstacles at home, in your relationships, or at work. You

may find yourself moving past obstacles as opposed to being stopped by them. This is the shift in mental clarity and empowerment that I have referred to on numerous occasions.

Center and Balance

This exercise system requires a tremendous amount of attention to being anchored within your center. As your opposing body parts move in opposition, to be physically stable you will have to engage your core muscles. These include primarily your entire abdominal region, buttocks, lower back, and inner thighs. They will be working very hard in each and every exercise. As a result, your core muscles will become much stronger every time you participate in the 2-in-1 strength training system. As your core muscles become stronger, your balance will improve dramatically. Strengthening your core muscle groups will also help improve your posture and reduce, or even eliminate, any lower back pain you may have. I want you to pay close attention to, and make detailed observations of, your sense of center and balance.

Present

You cannot be present in the moment without being *centered* and *balanced*. You will have the opportunity to use each of your 2-in-1 workouts as a workshop in being present. I want you to really be "in the moment" while you are performing these exercises. It doesn't matter what degree of mastery you have over the exercises, but they should never become an unconscious or mindless activity. You should never just go through the motions. If you are looking ahead to the next exercise or allow your mind to stray from what you are doing, you will risk injuring yourself. Make it a point to focus on each muscle, what it's doing and how it feels. As these workouts become second nature, your ability to remain present throughout your day will improve. This is truly the secret of success, and when it is incorporated into your "real" life, it can lead to remarkable life changes.

As these routines become a part of your life, you will find that your body/mind awareness is present in longer and longer stretches during each session. This will soon translate into being more passionate and engaged for longer and longer stretches of your day. Whether you will experience this as an improvement in your libido or your attitude, or just as a certain swagger in your walk, I cannot predict. Be assured that when you enter a room you will bring with you a certain presence. If and when you notice this happening, take the time to make a note of it.

Goals

Working toward a goal will develop all of these power tools. You must always have an agenda, and you must strive to meet your fitness goals every day. When you create an ultimate goal and a date by which you want to achieve that goal, these personal commitments force you to become accountable. You must create an agenda so that you can meet all of your short-term or weekly goals. By mapping out your transformation in such a way, you will provide yourself with a concise game plan with clear objectives for success.

Your goal is clear. The next chapter will take all the guesswork out of the path you should take to reach that goal. I have created a simple format for you in the next chapter so that you can look at where you are right this very moment and plan out exactly what you need to do today to meet your short-term goals and, ultimately, reach your destination.

WEEKLY 2-IN-1 EXERCISE CHART					
	Sedentary	Beginning	Intermediate	Advanced	Extreme
Ages 20–30	4 10s	3 10s 2 20s	1 10 3 20s 1 30	1 10 3 20s 2 30s	3 20s 3 30s
Ages 30–40	3 10s	3 10s 1 20	2 10s 2 20s	1 10 2 20s 2 30s	1 10 3 20s 2 30s
Ages 40–50	2 10s	3 10s	3 10s 1 20	3 10s 2 20s	1 10 2 20s 1 30
Ages 50+	2 10s	3 10s	3 10s 1 20	3 10s 1 20	1 10 1 20 1 30

DR

CHAPTER SEVEN

READY, SET, GO!

Here is where we put it all together. Over the past several chapters, I have done everything in my power to motivate you, obtain a commitment from you, empower you, and provide you with all the knowledge and tools needed to reach your goal. You now understand how important your jour-

nal and calendar are to your overall success. You understand that in the end this is a body makeover along with a lifestyle transformation that will provide you innumerable benefits for life. You have learned how this revolutionary, proven training system, which includes Fat-Blasting Nutrition, Superfast Sculpting, and 2-in-1 Strength Training, will help you achieve your ultimate goal as efficiently as possible. You now have everything you need to succeed.

It's time to discuss the amount of work you are going to be doing to attain your goal. I will also discuss modifications to the 2-in-1 Strength Training exercises for those of you who have physical limitations that prevent you from performing certain movements. I will also discuss the reward system you will be using that will add a dimension of excitement to this program. I believe in rewarding oneself along the way, and I have outlined a way to do so.

In essence, you may have any or all of three primary goals. You may want to reduce body fat and trim down; you may want to tone and sculpt your muscles; or you may want to add bulk or muscle size. You may also want to do a

combination of all three, which is often the case. However, I want you to choose your top priority right now and make that your number one goal. Then choose your second and third goals in descending order. The reason is that each of these goals has a specific strategy.

You have reviewed the cardio chart and the strength training chart in the previous chapters. These charts are meant to be guidelines to follow, but they are not black-and-white rules. They contain the minimum cardio and strength training sessions you need to do based upon your age, fitness level, and goal to achieve success. This is where you can get creative and make this more fun than any of your previous exercise regimes. Based on your goals, desire, and time frame, you can choose to work harder at cardio exercise or strength training. You might prefer to do more cardio exercise than the cardio chart designates for your goal but not increase the number of strength routines you do per week—or vice versa.

Another consideration is the amount of time you remain at each level. If you begin exercising from the sedentary level, at some point you are going to progress to the beginning, then to the intermediate, and so on. I typically suggest a maximum of six weeks before advancing to the next level, but it really depends upon you and how quickly your body responds to both cardio exercise and the 2-in-1 Strength Training exercises. You may already be on a consistent cardio exercise routine, but realize that it's time to add in the strength training component. Or you may be strength training, but doing little or no cardio exercise. Again, this is where the fun begins. *You* can choose when to advance to the next level, based upon how comfortable you feel with your current level. You may also find that you progress quickly with the 2-in-1 Strength Training exercises but find that the cardio exercise is a little more challenging. The Body Express training system will give you the flexibility to formulate the exercise regime that works best for you.

When is it time to move up? That's a good question. The answer is "when you feel you are ready for additional work in a certain area." However, to see results continually, you will need to raise the bar continually. In other words, you will want to work progressively harder and harder until you reach your maintenance stage. For some of you, this might be four to six weeks; for others it might be several months. It really does not matter how long it takes you as long as you continually push yourself to work harder. What matters is that you don't get frustrated, complacent, or lazy throughout the process. You need to continually push yourself to greater and greater limits until you reach your ultimate goal, which should be maintenance level. You may progress to the intermediate level by the time you reach your goal. Once at this level it is

okay to stay there as long as you are still being challenged.

Fat Loss

To shed excess fat and lose inches, you must pay extra close attention to your Fat-Blasting Nutrition program because eating poorly is most likely the reason you need to lose body fat in the first place. Have you had a poor diet for a period of time? Adhering to your nutrition program will be a very important factor in your physical transformation. In addition to this new eating program, you must also pay close attention to your cardio exercise sessions.

Even if you are just beginning an exercise regimen and are finding it a little difficult, do your best to extend the duration of your cardio sessions by three to five minutes every couple of cardio sessions until your uninterrupted cardio activity meets the cardio chart guidelines. Also, remember you can break up your cardio exercise into ten-minute sessions if you need to. As you increase the length of each session, make adjustments to the intensity of your cardiovascular routine as well. Vary your routine by using intervals one day, Burst Cardio the next, perhaps the 100s the day after. By continually raising the bar, you will force your body to work harder, which will cause it to change. Shocking the body is key for change and results. Not only will your heart health improve rapidly, but you will also discover that the cardio sessions are your most useful tool in burning off excess fat. If you cannot commit to your cardio exercise for whatever reason, you will have a very hard time reaching your body-fat reduction goal.

The 2-in-1 workouts are very important regardless of how much weight you need to lose. If you have 50-plus pounds to lose, I guarantee that you will see incredible changes if you just follow the cardio and 2-in-1 exercise prescription provided by the charts. For you, adding lean muscle mass is critical to kick-start your metabolism into high gear and enable you to burn more calories throughout the day. You also need to improve your cardio stamina and endurance so that you can eventually complete every exercise routine in the shortest time. In short, by eating regularly and properly, you will control your caloric intake, and by expending more calories through aerobic and strength training exercise, you will melt away the excess pounds while improving your cardio output and adding lean muscle mass.

Toning and Sculpting

If your goal is to tone, shape, and sculpt your muscles, your strategy will be similar to that of those who want to lose weight. To gain more definition, you will need to make sure you adhere very closely to the Fat-Blasting Nutrition strategy, have a solid cardio routine, and consistently do the 2-in-1 Strength Training exercises. Of primary importance will be your 2-in-1 Strength Training routine.

I am going to assume that you have only 5 to 25 pounds of excess body fat to lose, which is precisely why a sculpted body is within close reach. If your nutrition strategy and cardio exercise are consistent and burning off excess fat as they should, the 2-in-1 Strength Training routines will play a major role in rapidly sculpting your body. You may want to add an additional day or two of strength training with the 10, 20,

or 30 Routines. You will need to make sure that you move from one exercise to another as quickly as possible. Being able to go from one exercise to another with very little, if any, rest is the optimal way to work each strength routine. If you are not ready for that much work, pace yourself and work up to it. Your goal should be to do these exercises in rapid succession.

Building Lean Muscle Mass

If your ultimate goal is to increase lean muscle mass or add bulk or size, the 2-in-1 exercises will help you achieve that goal. Your Fat-Blasting Nutrition strategy and Superfast Sculpting cardio sessions will still be vital; however, the focus should be on the 2-in-1 exercise routines. You will want to add extra 10, 20, or 30 Routines into your week, working at a pace that is realistic yet pushes you. You will also want to gradually increase the weight you are using, which is the key in adding size. You will save yourself hours in the gym each day and still achieve the same, or even better, results in less than thirty minutes per workout.

Additionally, if building lean muscle mass or bulk is of primary importance, recovery time is also important. To give yourself enough recovery time, I suggest not doing the 30 Routine on back-to-back days. Mix in a 10 or 20 Routine between the days when you do the 30 Routine. I have structured each routine to be a total-body workout, so you will work each muscle group hard, but not to complete failure. This will allow you to train the same muscle groups on consecutive days by mixing in the 10 and 20 Routines with the 30 Routine.

These revolutionary workouts were designed to completely work several body parts simultaneously, and as a result they are the most time-efficient strength training system ever created. Instead of thirty minutes in a gym, you can do ten minutes at home. Instead of wasting an hour of waiting to use machines in a gym, you can accomplish the same result in twenty minutes in your living room. Instead of spending an hour with a personal trainer, you can get the same results in just thirty minutes without ever leaving your home.

Modifications

There are modifications for the 10, 20, and 30 Routines for individuals who are extremely overweight (obese) or out of shape or who have medical issues that limit their mobility. I have sometimes had to make modifications for certain clients. If the exercises in the 10, 20, and 30 Routines are too difficult to complete due to one of the above factors, all you have to do is scale them back a little.

The way to do this is by performing only one primary exercise at a time and then doing the secondary exercise by itself. The primary exercise is always the first exercise listed. If necessary, you can even do many of the exercises in a seated position. Granted, it will take you a little longer to complete each routine, but you will still see amazing results. For instance, if I have you holding a lunge, while performing an arm exercise such as biceps curls or lateral raises, simply perform each exercise separately. For instance, you can perform the biceps curls in a sitting or standing position and then hold the lunge for one minute. If you are doing a floor exercise such as lateral leg raises with rear raises, do the lateral leg raises first, then do the rear raises immediately afterward. Similarly, if you are doing an abdominal exercise with a secondary movement, I would suggest doing the abdominal exercise first, then the secondary movement.

If an exercise calls for some form of lunge or squat, I want you to go only as low as is comfortable for you, or do your squats with a big ball behind you against a wall. As you get stronger and develop stamina, endurance, and a better sense of balance, you will be able to go lower into these exercises. The key is to start slowly and work yourself up to a point where you can perform both components of each exercise simultaneously. There is no judgment here. Everyone has to start from somewhere, and that starting point will be determined by you and directly related to your current physical condition. In time you will be able to do each exercise and routine as they were designed to be done, unless you have a physical disability, in which case you will do each routine to the best of your physical ability.

Don't let the difficulty of these exercises stop you from becoming the *you* you want to be. Don't let any disadvantages you may have prevent you from achieving your dream body. We all have obstacles to face. These obstacles are greater for some of us than for others. I absolutely understand your fear of failure and your concern that you might hurt yourself in some way. If you are very weak, a little uncoordinated, or disadvantaged in any way, take it easy and do one exercise at a time. It may take you a little longer to reach your goals, but you will reach them if you really put your heart, soul, and trust into the process. I know it works; I have proven it time and again.

Stabilization, Balance, and Core

You are probably reading through this book as fast as possible so you can get started on your Body Express Makeover and I encourage you to do so. However, for those of you who are over 50 years of age, have prior injuries, have been sedentary for a long period of time, or who may be extremely overweight, I have one additional recommendation. The Body Express 2-in-1 exercises are not only multi–muscle group exercises—they also require a certain degree of balance and core strength to be done properly. This is because several exercises include lunge and squat motions, martial arts stances and kicks, along with yoga postures. Although I demonstrated in the modifications section how most exercises can be made easier, I would suggest some additional balance and core strength work for those of you who fit the above criteria.

It's important to understand that your body consists of a kinetic chain that is linked together. This chain is comprised of the nervous system, the skeletal system, and the muscular system. All three systems need to work in unison for optimal performance. In other words, we want all three systems to communicate optimally for neuromuscular efficiency. This means that when your nervous system (your brain) sends nerve impulses to the skeletal system to bend over, turn sideways, or jump over an obstacle, it's important that the right muscles are recruited in the right order with the right nerve impulses. It's very much like having the right directions to a location. If the directions are wrong it will be difficult to arrive at your destination. We develop this neuromuscular efficiency by strengthening the core in both stable and unstable environments. In doing so we will also reduce the time it will take you to reach your ultimate goal. If you fit any of the categories I mentioned above, I would suggest doing a few of the following exercises.

For one to two weeks prior to beginning the 2-in-1 Strength Training exercises I would like you to partake in a few balance and core strengthening exercises as a foundation for the actual 2-in-1 programs. During this time I still want you to follow the Fat-Blasting nutritional strategy, the Superfast Sculpting cardio exercise, and the flexibility programs you will read about later in chapter 11. Developing this balance and core foundation will greatly improve your ability to do the 2-in-1 exercises properly and will also reduce any chance of injury. The idea is for you to succeed in reaching your ultimate goal, but also to do so with the proper body mechanics.

These five exercises can also be done concurrently with the 2-in-1 Strength Training routines. These are exercises you can do for the rest of your life to ensure that you are properly utilizing your core and continue to improve your balance and coordination. Practicing these exercises as prescribed will increase your core strength and improve the communication between your nervous, skeletal, and muscular systems. This in turn will ensure that you are on track to achieve the results you are looking for and to have the body you have always dreamed about having.

■■■

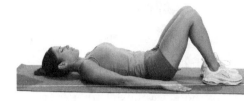

Figure 1

In this first core strengthening exercise, I would like you to lie on a mat on your back with your knees bent and feet pointed straight ahead directly under your knees with hands by your sides, palms facing downward (Figure 1). In this position rotate your pelvis backward creating a slight arch in your back and then rotate your pelvis forward creating a concave curve in your back. From here I want you to rotate your pelvis such that it is exactly in the middle or what we refer to as neutral position. Then slowly, to the count of four, arch and bring your pelvis up as high as comfortable, hold for 2 counts, and then release back down for 2 counts. Do 2 sets of 12 repetitions 3 to 5 days a week until you feel that your core is stronger. Make sure your knees

do not buckle inward. If they do, put a small medicine ball between them to prevent them from doing so. On the flip side if your knees bow outward, wrap a band around them to prevent them from doing so. By constricting your knee movement you will reeducate your body to do this exercise correctly and strengthen your core.

In this second exercise, you will still be on the mat, but this time you will lie on your stomach with

your hands by your side, palms facing downward. This is the precursor exercise to the Superman stretch you will find in chapter 11 on flexibility. Slowly, to a count of four, raise your upper torso upward as high as you feel comfortable, squeezing your shoulder blades together as you do so. Hold for 2 counts and release down for 2 counts. Perform 2 sets of 12 repetitions 3 to 5 days a week to strengthen your mid and lower back.

For this third exercise, you will stand tall with your feet pointing straight ahead directly under your shoulders (Figure 2). Once again do the forward and backward pelvis rotations to find neutral position. From here I want you to raise one foot about 12 inches off the floor and point your toe to your shin. Feel free to use a chair to balance yourself if necessary. Hold this position for 15 seconds and then repeat on the other foot. It's important to hold your pelvis in a neutral position and engage your abdominal area for support. Do 2 sets of 12 repetitions, 6 on each foot, 3 to 5 days a week until you can hold each foot off the ground for 30 seconds without difficulty. This exercise will strengthen your core and balance.

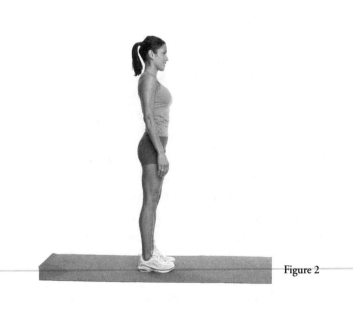

Figure 2

In this fourth exercise, from the same standing position (Figure 3), raise one foot about 12 inches off the floor, hold your balance, and then hop from one side to the other, alternating the landing foot. Use a chair for balance if necessary. Hold the landing position for 5 seconds and then hop back onto the other foot. It's not about how high you jump, it's about keeping that neutral pelvis position and keeping the abdominals engaged. Do 2 sets of 12 hops, 6 on each side, 3 to 5 days a week. Once this exercise begins to get easy due to increased core strength, you can begin the progression of allowing your body to lower down into a one-legged squat while holding that neutral position. This exercise will strengthen your core and balance.

For this fifth and final exercise, you will start from the same standing position. Find your neutral pelvic position and slowly step out with one foot into a down lunge position, making sure that your front heel is directly in alignment with your front knee (Figure 4). Only go down as far as you feel comfortable. In time, as your core and leg strength increases, you will be able to go lower to the ground. Hold the lunge for 20 to 30 seconds and then repeat on the other side. Perform 2 sets of 12 repetitions, 6 for each leg, 3 to 5 times per day.

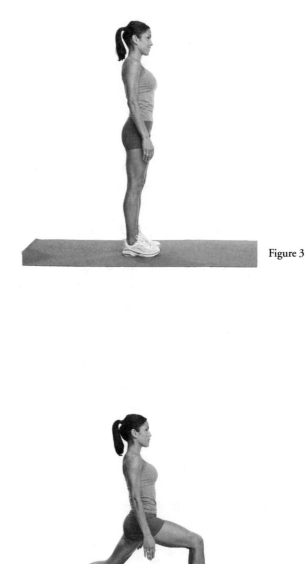

Figure 3

Figure 4

Designing Your Exercise Routine

If you follow the 2-in-1 Strength Training routines, you will rapidly see amazing results in your muscle strength, endurance, and tone. However, it is important to understand that at some point your body may get used to doing the exercises in each routine if you do them with the same amount of weight and in the same order over a period of time.

The key to continually realizing results is to continually shock your muscles by placing them under greater stress. You can do this by gradually increasing the weight you are using and decreasing the rest time between exercises, therefore increasing the intensity while still being safe. At some point you may hit a plateau and find that your muscles no longer respond as quickly as before. To overcome this plateau, I suggest mixing up the exercises by changing the order in which you do them. Always start with the first exercise in each routine because it is a warm-up exercise, but feel free to perform the remaining ones in whichever order you'd like. This will shock your muscles, and you will kickstart new muscle development.

Another great feature of the 2-in-1 exercise routines is that you can customize each exercise by doing different secondary exercises with each primary exercise. This is another way to shock your muscles. This can be done very easily but will take some creativity on your part. For instance, if one exercise calls for a ball squat with shoulder presses and another calls for a lunge hold with biceps curls, all you have to do is switch the two arm exercises. Another example would be if one exercise calls for a closed T stance with lateral raises and another calls for a lunge hold with double triceps kickbacks, once again you could switch the arm exercises. Not every exercise can be altered creatively, but enough of them can be changed to give you a number of different options. In essence, you will be able to change each routine enough to shock your body into muscle hypertrophy, which is an increase in muscle fiber and strength.

Reward System

Here is the fun part. I use a reward system with my clients because it helps them to be more accountable both to themselves and to me as their trainer. I want you to use a reward system too. If you know that you are going to receive a reward every few weeks for putting in the effort to be consistent with the Body Express Makeover training system, you will find it much more motivating and fun. Remember back in grade school when you finished a project and did a good job on it, your teacher would give you a gold star or sometimes a piece of candy? Remember how happy and proud you felt for getting that prize? Remember how hard you worked to get that reward? The same thing works when it comes to eating healthfully and exercising. In the workplace, many of us receive bonuses for some reason, whether a year-end bonus or a bonus for finishing a project. Many salespeople receive commissions in addition to their salary. These are all forms of a reward system and are in place to push us all to work harder to reach our goals. Reward systems work very well, and it's the reason I use them, successfully, with my clients.

We always feel great when we go out and purchase something nice for ourselves, but it means even more when we know we've worked hard and deserve it. Deserving the reward is what this reward system is all about, so I'm asking you to be very honest with yourself. There is a fine line between expecting more from yourself and being overly critical of yourself, and I want you to pay close attention to it. Don't give yourself a reward if you didn't earn it, but at the same time don't set unrealistic goals so that you never have the opportunity to reward yourself. I've purposely left room for individual interpretation in the reward system, so it will be up to you to make ongoing, conscious decisions about how well you are adhering to your makeover and lifestyle transformation.

The first six weeks of this new way of eating and exercising will likely be the most challenging period. After those initial six weeks, you will have successfully made this new lifestyle a habit that you will keep for life. To make the first six weeks a little easier, I want you to reward yourself at the end of every two-week period. If you can adhere to your new nutrition strategy and exercise program four out of seven days for the first two weeks, give yourself an inexpensive gift. It might be a manicure, a new CD or DVD, or a night out at the movies. For the next two weeks, strive to adhere to the nutrition and exercise program five out of seven days. If you accomplish this goal, reward yourself with something a little more special. Maybe it will be a spa day, a new pair of shoes, or a nice pair of slacks—now one size smaller! It might be a day spent participating in an activity that you love but don't normally allow yourself the luxury of time to do. For the last two weeks, strive to be consistent with your program at least six days each week. If you achieve this goal, congratulate yourself for

sticking to your commitment with an even bigger reward, maybe a weekend away, new golf clubs, or that new Prada purse you've been wanting.

The key is to make sure each reward is a little better than the last. It's also important to remember that your rewards don't always have to be of monetary value. Take a break from housework and read a book, go visit a friend whom you haven't seen in a while, or spend a leisurely day at the beach or park. Our busy lives often prevent us from taking time to relax and enjoy the world around us. I want you to really reward yourself by doing something you never get to do, whether it costs $500 or absolutely nothing.

Now open your journal to the "Notes to Self" section and write down the three rewards you will give yourself. Be creative. It's important to write them down in advance so you know what you will receive prior to successfully achieving each and every two-week goal. Just like professional athletes or top salespeople, you will spend countless hours honing your skills for a reward that is known to you beforehand. For them the reward might be a medal, a trophy, or a ring, but knowing what they are striving for in advance motivates them to succeed, and it will motivate you too.

After the initial six weeks, I want you to begin your reward system again, with different rewards. From this point on, I want you to structure your reward system so that you get a reward every four weeks. I would like you to continue this reward system, or at least a scaled-down version of it, for the rest of your life. The reason is that having a reward system in place is a very powerful tool in keeping you consistently accountable to yourself. You will continually recognize your efforts and how well you are adhering to this new lifestyle. By doing so, you will greatly reduce the chance that you will stray from your new, healthy lifestyle for extended periods of time. The important thing is to be present in the moment. When you get complacent and lose sight of the present, you find yourself out of balance and your priorities begin to get jumbled and juxtaposed. That's exactly what you want to avoid.

This state of awareness is where I would like you to remain throughout your life. Being consistent with your new nutrition plan and exercise regime 90 percent of the time is a very realistic and achievable goal. It also allows you to be human. Throughout this book I have emphasized the importance of setting realistic goals. This also means living a realistic lifestyle that allows for social events, holidays, lack of planning, and little slips. We are human, and we get lazy, bored, and complacent at times. But beating ourselves up and engaging in self-defeating behavior is counterproductive. We need to acknowledge and understand what makes us do what we do. Knowing what triggers you to overeat in the afternoon or skip a workout will help you figure out a way to prevent it in the future. I can almost certainly predict that most of these occurrences are caused by lack of planning, so be aware of this. Use your calendar religiously, and plan for every possible disruption.

We as a society love to celebrate almost any occasion: birthdays, holidays, graduations, marriages, a new baby, a promotion, you name it. Celebrating is one of the ways in which we connect with friends and family. It provides us with joy and an escape from the grind of daily life. There is nothing wrong with having a piece of birthday cake or missing a couple days of exercise due to life events, whether joyous or crisis. The key is to make sure that these account for only 10 percent of your time, or as close to that figure as possible. This is what we call moderation. If you adhere to your new lifestyle 90 percent of the time, you can easily afford to indulge yourself 10 percent of the time. That's why you will find it so easy and simple to adhere to the Body Express Makeover system: it allows you to live life without deprivation. Living a healthy lifestyle is not about being perfect; it's about striving to be the healthiest you can be on any given day.

Have fun with yourself, your new body, and your new lifestyle and see what rewards they bring you. One of the greatest gifts you can give to friends and loved ones is a healthy, happy you. Imagine how happy they will be when you are taking care of yourself and living a positive, healthy life. Pass along the message of healthy living to others, and see what gifts come back to you.

Now it's time to review the exercise and flexibility routines and get started on your body makeover.

CHAPTER EIGHT

THE 10 ROUTINE

During the 10 Routine you will perform only one set of each exercise. Do your utmost to complete each exercise as best you can. Make sure to always do some form of light warm-up activity for at least ten minutes prior to doing any form of exercise and also ten minutes of cool down after exercising. Work through the routine as quickly as you can—pushing yourself, but not so hard that you risk injury. Do each exercise fully throughout a complete range of motion. The goal here is to complete the 10 Routine as quickly as you can so as to keep your heart rate up and burn more calories. If you need to rest, the optimal rest time is thirty seconds to one minute, but strive to stay within this time frame. Each exercise has a modification so that you can work up to completing each exercise as it was designed. Have fun with this routine, as it will become a staple of your exercise program.

For the first six weeks, I recommend you follow the routine for your gender only in the exact order shown here. When you are familiar with your gender's routines, you can customize your workout if you feel a particular exercise better targets an area of the body you wish to focus on. It is important to note that you don't need to customize any of the exercises or routines to meet your goals.

10 ROUTINE

Female	10 Exercises/1 Set Each	Male	10 Exercises/1 Set Each
1 set of 5 reps	Sun Salutation w/Two Push-ups	1 set of 15 reps	Squat Thrust w/Push-up
1 set of 20 reps	Ab Crunch w/Inner Thigh Squeeze (weighted ball)	1 set of 20 reps	Ab Crunch (Legs Up) w/Reverse Crunch
1 set of 20 reps	George's Oblique w/Inner Thigh Pulse (ankle weights)	1 set of 20 reps	Ball Crunch w/Chest Press
1 set of 20 reps	Glute Kickback w/ Opposite Triceps Kickback (ankle weights)	1 set of 20 reps	Alternating Lunge w/Shoulder Press
1 set of 20 reps	Bench Dip w/Alternating Leg Extension (ankle weights)	1 set of 20 reps	Ball Chest Fly w/Double Triceps Extension
1 set of 20 reps	Standing Side Leg Raise w/One-Arm Side Lateral Raise (ankle weights)	1 set of 20 reps	Squat and Calf Raise w/Biceps Curl
1 set of 20 reps	Wall Sit w/Shoulder Press	1 set of 20 reps	Single Arm Row w/Reverse Triceps Kickback
1 set of 20 reps	Left Lunge Hold w/Double Triceps Extension	1 set of 20 reps	Right Lunge Hold w/Side Lateral Raise
1 set of 20 reps	Right Lunge Hold w/Front Lateral Raise	1 set of 20 reps	Left Lunge Hold w/Biceps Curl
1 set of 20 reps	Plié Squat and Calf Raise w/Biceps Curl	1 set of 20 reps	Wall Sit w/Front Lateral Raise

sun salutation with two push-ups (female)

READY: Core, chest, shoulders, triceps, lower back, quadriceps, hamstrings, gluteus maximus, and outer thighs

SET: Stand with your feet shoulder width apart and your arms by your sides (Figure 5).

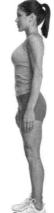

Figure 5

GO: Inhale, turn your arms outward so your palms face out, lift your arms up and out to each side in an arclike motion, and bring your arms over your head, reaching and lengthening as you go. At the top of the movement, your palms will meet in a "praying hands" position (Figure 6).

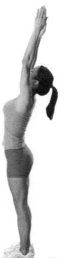

Figure 6

Exhale, bend at the waist, and lower the upper half of your body until your palms rest on the ground (Figure 7).

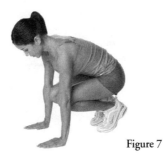

Figure 7

Step or jump your feet back into the push-up position (Figure 8). Perform two push-ups. Hold for a beat, then raise your hips upward until your body resembles an inverted "V" with your buttocks pointing upward. Push back on your heels (Figure 9). (In yoga, this is the Downward Dog.) Lower your hips until you are back in the plank or push-up position (Figure 8).

Do two push-ups (Figure 10).

modification: You can do the push-ups on your knees or leave them out completely until you are strong enough to do them.

At the bottom of the second push-up, arch up with the crown of your head leading the way, and raise your head upward, looking straight ahead and trying to keep your thighs off the floor (Figure 11). (In yoga, this is the Upward Dog.)

modification: You can lower your thighs to the floor.

Push back into the plank position (Figure 10) and then up, raising your buttocks upward while pushing yourself back into the Downward Dog position (Figure 9). Step or jump your feet back toward your hands and then roll back up, lengthening your spine, until you are back in the standing position (Figure 12). Stand tall and repeat.

1 set of 5 repetitions

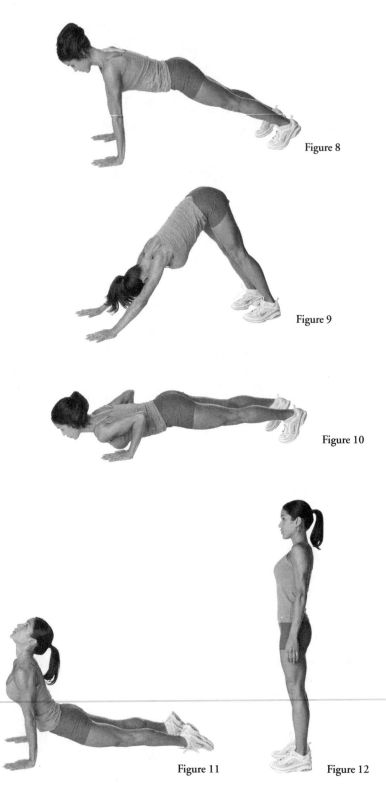

Figure 8

Figure 9

Figure 10

Figure 11

Figure 12

squat thrust with push-up (male)

READY: Core, chest, shoulders, triceps, lower back, quadriceps, hamstrings, gluteus maximus, and outer thighs

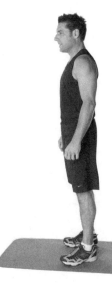

SET: Stand with your hands by your sides (Figure 13).

Figure 13

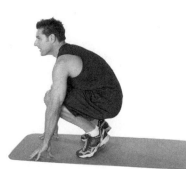

GO: Bend at the waist, and lower the upper half of your body down until your fingertips rest on the ground (Figure 14). Jump your feet back so you are in a plank or push-up position (Figure 15).

Figure 14

Do a push-up, keeping your lower back straight, pushing back with your heels, and lowering your chest close to the ground (Figure 16). Come back up until your elbows lock (Figure 15).

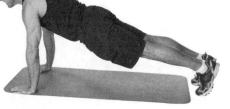

modification: You can do these push-ups on your knees.

Figure 15

Jump your feet to your hands and stand up tall (Figures 14 and 13).

1 set of 15 repetitions

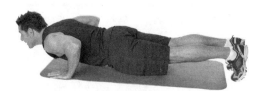

Figure 16

abdominal crunch with inner thigh squeeze (with weighted ball) (female)

READY: core, upper and mid abdominals, and inner thighs

Although a weighted ball is preferred, you can use any ball, such as a basketball, a volleyball, a soccer ball, or even a tennis ball. Just make sure that the ball has enough "give" that it can be squeezed.

SET: Lie on your back with your feet on the ground and your legs bent. Place the ball between your knees. Join your hands behind your head (Figure 17).

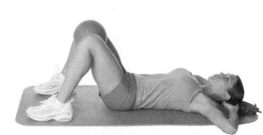

Figure 17

GO: Raise your shoulders off the floor, coming up into a crunch. Make sure to use your abdominal muscles, not your neck, to come up into the crunch (Figure 18).

simultaneously:

Squeeze your thighs together. Release down slowly.

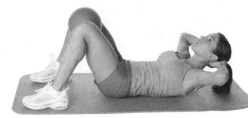

Figure 18

modification: Raise your shoulders off the floor only as far as is comfortable. After a while your abdominals will become stronger and you will be able to come up higher.

1 set of 20 repetitions

abdominal crunch (legs up) with reverse crunch (male)

READY: Core; upper and lower abdominals

SET: Lie on your back with your knees bent. Raise your feet upward until your thighs are perpendicular to the floor, your knees still bent. Cross your ankles and join your hands behind your head (Figure 19).

GO: Raise your shoulders off the floor, coming up into a crunch (Figure 20). Release your upper torso back down to the start position. Then, using your lower abdominals, lift your buttocks off the ground 1 to 2 inches, raising your knees upward and trying not to swing your legs for momentum (Figure 21).

modification: For the reverse crunch, you can lower your legs so your knees are right above your stomach. Then raise your knees toward your chest. Do this until your lower abs are strong enough to do the original version.

1 set of 20 repetitions

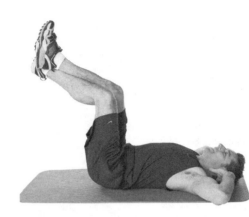

Figure 19

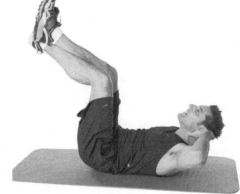

Figure 20

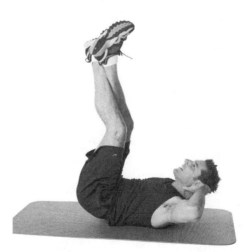

Figure 21

george's oblique with inner thigh pulse (with ankle weights) (female)

READY: Core, abdominals, obliques, and inner thighs

SET: Put on a pair of 3- to 5-pound ankle weights. Lie on your back and extend your left leg. Bring your right leg over the left and place your right foot flat on the ground, outside your left knee. You are now balancing somewhat on your left buttock. Your right hand is behind your head; your left arm is across your waist (Figure 22).

modification: Your left hand can rest on the floor beside your torso for support.

GO: Bring your right elbow up toward your right knee, without snapping your neck, and raise your left leg as high as you can (Figure 23).

modification: You can do this without ankle weights or with lighter ankle weights. You can also do one exercise at a time.

Release back down to the start position and repeat the exercise. Then switch to the other side and repeat.

1 set of 20 repetitions on both sides

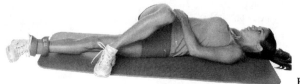

Figure 22

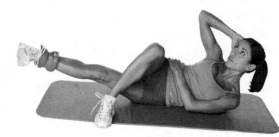

Figure 23

ball crunch with chest press (male)

READY: Core, chest, upper and mid abdominals, lower back, and quadriceps

SET: Sit on a therapy ball with a dumbbell in each hand. Roll back so that the ball is under your lower to mid back. Position the dumbbells on the same plane as your shoulders. (If you were holding a barbell, it would be lying on top of your collarbone.)

Raise your head and tuck your chin, creating abdominal tension (Figure 24).

GO: Raise your shoulders off the ball into a crunch.

simultaneously:

Push the dumbbells up directly over your chest. Bring them together and squeeze your chest together. Hold for a beat (Figure 25).

modification: If you have a neck injury or weak abdominals, roll out on the ball until your neck is resting on the ball and use lighter hand weights (Figure 26). Do the chest press first, and then do the abdominal crunches on the ball separately until you are strong enough to do both together.

Return to the start position.

1 set of 20 repetitions

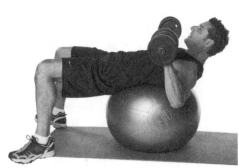

Figure 24

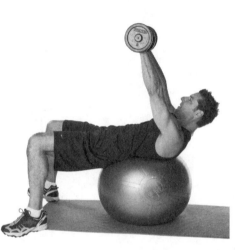

Figure 25

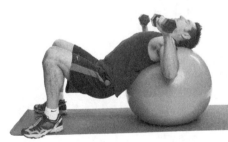

Figure 26

glute kickback with opposite triceps kickback (with ankle weight) (female)

READY: Core, gluteus maximus, hips, hamstrings, outer thighs, and triceps

SET: Put a 3- to 5-pound ankle weight on your left ankle and get onto your elbows and knees. Hold a dumbbell in your right hand and rest your body on your left forearm. Bring your right arm tight into your rib cage until your arm is in an inverted "V" position and your elbow is pointed upward (Figure 27).

GO: Extend your left leg back, pushing back with your heel, until your leg is fully extended and slightly higher than your torso.

simultaneously:

Using only the hinge of your elbow, extend the dumbbell backward until your right arm is fully extended (Figure 28). Release back into the start position. After you complete all the repetitions, switch sides.

modification: You can do this exercise without ankle weights. You can also do one exercise at a time until you are able to do both together.

1 set of 20 repetitions on both sides

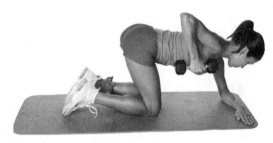

Figure 27

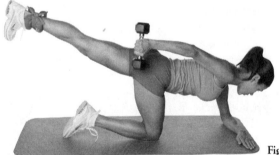

Figure 28

alternating lunge with shoulder press (male)

READY: Core, quadriceps, gluteus maximus, hamstrings, calves, inner thighs, shoulders, triceps, balance, and coordination

SET: Stand with a dumbbell in each hand. Bring the dumbbells up until they are aligned with your shoulders, keeping your upper arms against your rib cage, your palms facing forward (Figure 29).

GO: Step out with your left foot and go down into a lunge position, keeping your left knee in alignment with your left heel and your back straight.

simultaneously:

Press the dumbbells upward until your arms are almost locked (Figure 30). Lower your arms back into the start position as you step back into a standing position (Figure 29). Alternate legs until you complete all the repetitions.

modification: Do one exercise at a time and go down into the lunge only as far as is comfortable. In time your legs will be strong enough to go all the way down.

1 set of 20 repetitions

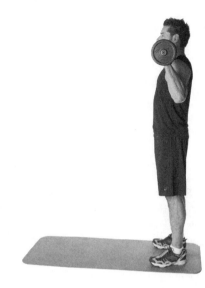

Figure 29

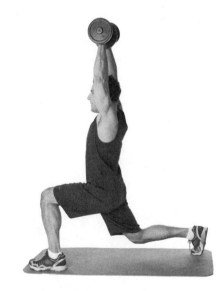

Figure 30

bench dip with alternating leg extension (with ankle weights) (female)

READY: Core, triceps, wrists, and quadriceps

SET: Put on pair of 5- to 10-pound ankle weights. Sit on a chair or bench. Place your palms on the seat of the chair, your fingers facing outward, and walk your feet out until they are in a 90-degree angle. Your arms are now supporting you (Figure 31).

GO: Bending only at your elbows, lower yourself until your arms are bent at a 90-degree angle and your upper arms are parallel to the ground.

simultaneously:

Extend your left leg outward, pushing out with the heel and keeping your left knee as high off the ground as possible (Figure 32). Push yourself back up to the start position as you place your left foot back on the ground. Repeat, but this time extend with your right leg. Continue alternating legs until the desired number of repetitions is completed.

modification: Lower yourself only as far as is comfortable. You can also do one exercise at a time.

1 set of 20 repetitions

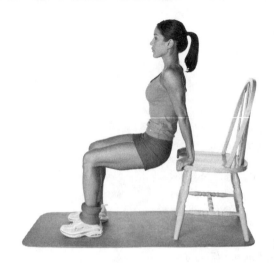

Figure 31

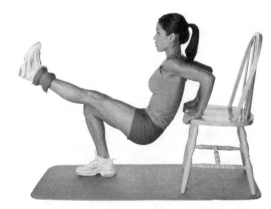

Figure 32

ball chest fly with double triceps extension (male)

READY: Core, abdominals, chest, and triceps

SET: With a dumbbell in each hand, sit on top of a therapy ball. Roll back so that the ball is underneath your lower back. Position the dumbbells so they are directly above your chest, your elbows slightly bent and your palms facing each other, as if you were hugging a barrel.

Raise up a little and tuck your chin in toward your chest, creating abdominal tension (Figure 33).

GO: Lower the dumbbells until your hands are in alignment with your shoulders, still keeping the elbows bent, releasing your upper torso (Figure 34). Push the dumbbells back up until the dumbbells almost touch. Hold for a beat as you squeeze your chest muscles together (Figure 35).

Using only the elbow joint as a hinge, lower the dumbbells toward your shoulder blades until only your elbows are pointed upward (Figure 36). Push the dumbbells back up until your arms are fully extended (Figure 35).

Repeat both exercises for the desired number of repetitions.

modification: If you have neck problems or a neck injury, roll out on the ball so that it is directly under your neck. You can also do one exercise at a time.

1 set of 20 repetitions

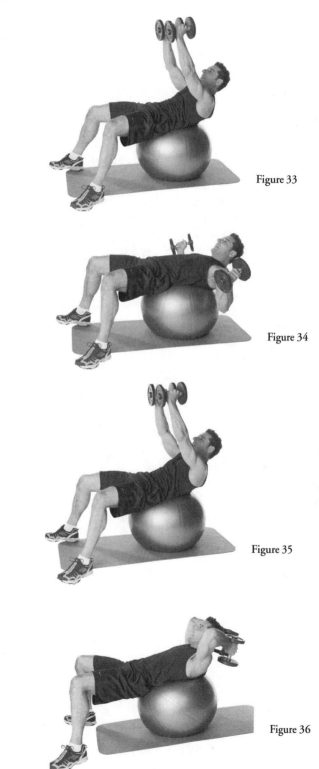

Figure 33

Figure 34

Figure 35

Figure 36

standing side leg raise with one-arm side lateral raise (with ankle weights) (female)

READY: Core, outer thighs, hips, and shoulders

SET: Put a 3- to 5-pound ankle weight on your left leg and hold a dumbbell in your left hand. Stand next to a chair or a wall that will support your weight. Hold on to the chair with your right hand and stand up tall.

GO: Bend your right knee slightly. Leading with your ankle, lift your left leg straight out to the side as high as you can. Keep your upper torso as straight as possible.

simultaneously:

Bend your left elbow slightly and lift your left arm straight out to the side until the dumbbell is at shoulder level (Figure 37). Release back down to the start position and complete repetitions. Then switch sides.

modification: Do only one exercise at a time.

1 set of 20 repetitions on both sides

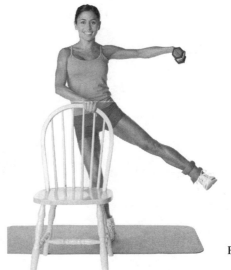

Figure 37

squat and calf raise with biceps curl (male)

READY: Core, quadriceps, hamstrings, gluteus maximus, outer thighs, calves, lower back, and biceps

SET: Stand with a dumbbell in each hand, your palms facing outward and your feet slightly wider than shoulder width apart, toes pointed slightly outward (Figure 38).

GO: Raise the dumbbells toward your shoulders in a curling motion, and at the top of the movement, twist your wrists slightly so the backs of your hands are directed toward each other, keeping your elbows tight into your rib cage.

simultaneously:

Arch your back slightly, keeping your upper torso over your pelvis, then lower yourself down as if you were sitting in a chair. Go down as far as is comfortable. As you get stronger, you will be able to go lower (Figure 39).

As you come back up, lower your arms to the start position and push your pelvis forward slightly; squeeze your gluteus maximus together, and raise up onto the balls of your feet in an explosive movement (Figure 40). Hold for a beat. Release back to the start position and repeat.

modification: You can do one exercise at a time.

1 set of 20 repetitions

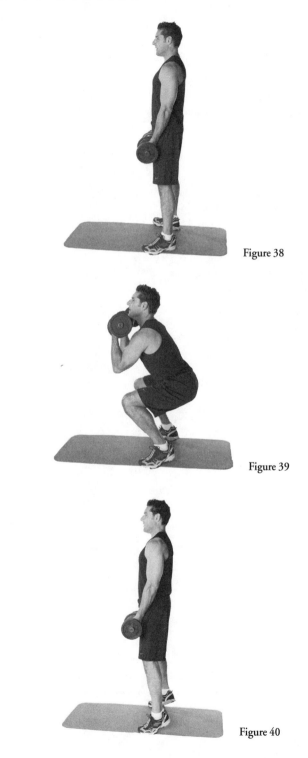

Figure 38

Figure 39

Figure 40

wall sit with shoulder press (female)

READY: Core, quadriceps, hamstrings, outer thighs, and shoulders

SET: With a dumbbell in each hand, stand against a wall. Walk your feet out and lower your buttocks until you look as though you are sitting in a chair (Figure 41).

GO: Extend your arms upward until they are fully extended, then lower them (Figure 42). Repeat.

modification: You may choose a less-than-seated position to make it easier.

Remain in this position throughout the exercise.

1 set of 20 repetitions

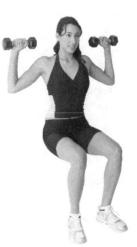

Figure 41

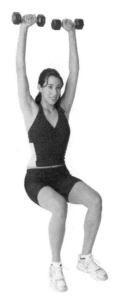

Figure 42

single arm row with reverse triceps kickback (male)

READY: Core, quadriceps, hamstrings, gluteus maximus, calves, back, and triceps

SET: Stand with a dumbbell in your right hand. Step forward with your left foot and drop down into a lunge position. Lean your torso slightly forward, place your left arm on top of your left leg, and arch your back slightly with your chest directly above your left thigh.

Remain in this position throughout the exercise.

GO: Extend your right arm below you with the dumbbell close to the floor and your palm facing backward (Figure 43). In a rowing motion, raise the dumbbell up, twisting your wrist so your palm turns toward your torso, until the dumbbell is even with your rib cage (Figure 44).

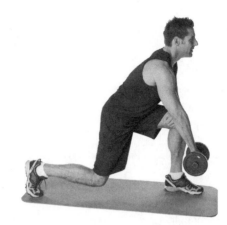

Figure 43

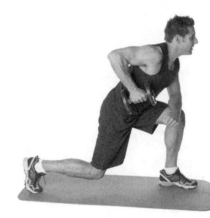

Figure 44

Using your elbow joint as a hinge, extend your right arm backward, leading with the heel of your hand, until your arm is fully extended (Figure 45). Hold for a beat; then unlock your elbow and release the dumbbell back down to the floor. Repeat until you complete the desired number of repetitions. Then switch sides.

modification: You can do one exercise at a time.

1 set of 20 repetitions on both sides

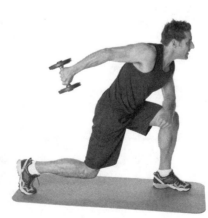

Figure 45

left lunge hold with double triceps extension (female)

READY: Core, quadriceps, hamstrings, gluteus maximus, calves, inner thighs, triceps, and balance

SET: Stand with a dumbbell in each hand.

Step forward with your left foot, pushing back with your right heel. Make sure your left knee is directly above your left heel and at a 90-degree angle. Lower yourself down only as far as comfortable from a strength standpoint.

Remain in this position throughout the exercise.

GO: Bring the dumbbells straight up above your head, directly above your shoulders, with your arms fully extended and your palms facing upward (Figure 46). Using only the elbow joint as a hinge, lower the dumbbells down toward your shoulder blades until your elbows are pointed upward (Figure 47). Push the dumbbells back up until your arms are fully extended (Figure 46) as you return to the start position. Repeat.

modification: Go down only as far as comfortable. You can also do one exercise at a time.

1 set of 20 repetitions

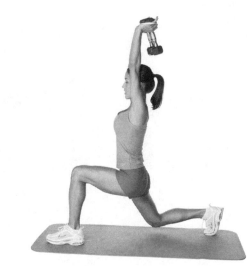

Figure 46

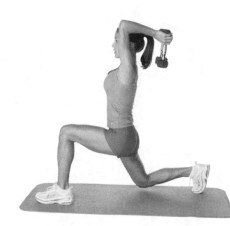

Figure 47

right lunge hold with side lateral raise (male)

READY: Core, quadriceps, gluteus maximus, hamstrings, calves, inner thighs, shoulders, and balance

SET: Stand with a dumbbell in each hand, your palms facing inward (Figure 48). Step forward with your right foot, lowering your left knee close to the floor. Make sure your left knee is directly above your right heel and at a 90-degree angle (Figure 49).

modification: Lower yourself only as far as is comfortable.

Remain in this position throughout the exercise.

GO: Bend your elbows slightly and raise your arms to the side, your palms pointing downward, until your arms come up to shoulder level (Figure 50). Lower your arms back into the start position (Figure 48).

1 set of 20 repetitions

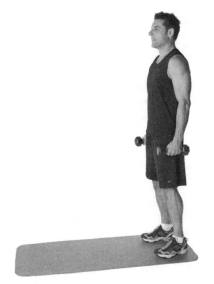

Figure 48

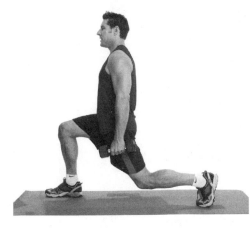

Figure 49

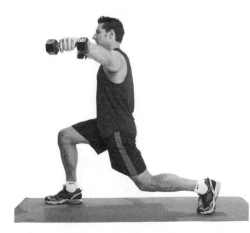

Figure 50

right lunge hold with front lateral raise (female)

READY: Core, quadriceps, gluteus maximus, hamstrings, calves, inner thighs, shoulders, and balance

SET: Stand with a dumbbell in each hand, your palms facing backward. Step forward with your right foot, lowering your left knee close to the floor. Make sure your right knee is directly above your right heel and at a 90-degree angle (Figure 51).

modification: Go down only as far as is comfortable until you are strong enough to go all the way down. You can also do one exercise at a time.

Remain in this position throughout the exercise.

GO: Bend your elbows slightly and raise your hands in front of you until the dumbbells come up to eye level (Figure 52). Lower your arms back to the start position (Figure 51).

1 set of 20 repetitions

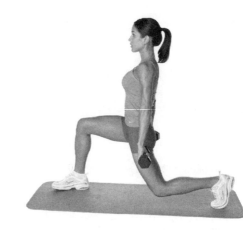

Figure 51

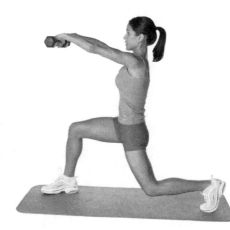

Figure 52

left lunge hold with biceps curl (male)

READY: Core, quadriceps, gluteus maximus, hamstrings, calves, inner thighs, biceps, and balance

SET: Stand with a dumbbell in each hand, your arms by your sides and your palms facing your torso. Step forward with your left foot, and lower your right knee close to the floor. Make sure your left knee is directly above your left heel and at a 90-degree angle (Figure 53).

modification: Go down only as far as is comfortable until you are strong enough to go all the way down. You can also do one exercise at a time.

Remain in this position throughout the exercise.

GO: Bring your arms up in a curling motion, and at the top of the movement, twist your wrists slightly so the backs of your hands are directed toward each other, keeping your elbows tight into your rib cage (Figure 54).

1 set of 20 repetitions

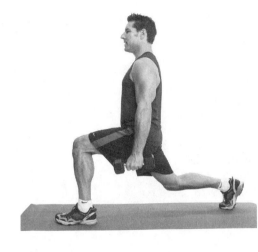

Figure 53

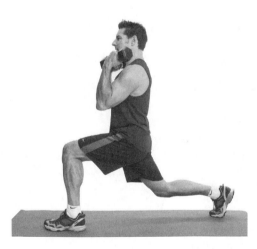

Figure 54

plié squat and calf raise with biceps curl (female)

READY: Core, quadriceps, hamstrings, gluteus maximus, outer and inner thighs, calves, lower back, and biceps

SET: Stand with a dumbbell in each hand and your palms facing forward, your feet slightly more than shoulder width apart and your toes pointed outward (Figure 55).

GO: Raise the dumbbells toward your shoulders in a curling motion. Turn the dumbbells outward at the top of the movement, keeping your elbows tight into your rib cage.

simultaneously:

Arch your back slightly, keeping your torso over your pelvis. Then lower yourself down as if you were sitting in a chair. Go down as far as is comfortable (Figure 56). As you get stronger, you will be able to go lower.

As you come back up, lower your arms to the start position, push your pelvis slightly forward, and squeeze your gluteus maximus together. Then raise up onto the balls of your feet in an explosive movement, contracting your calves (Figure 57). Hold for a beat. Release and return to the starting position (Figure 55).

modification: Go down only as far as is comfortable until you are strong enough to go all the way down. You can also do one exercise at a time.

1 set of 20 repetitions

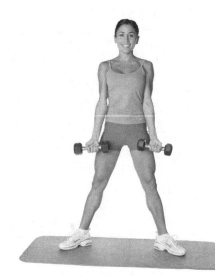

Figure 55

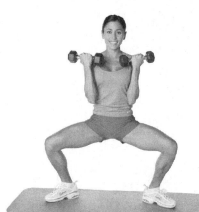

Figure 56

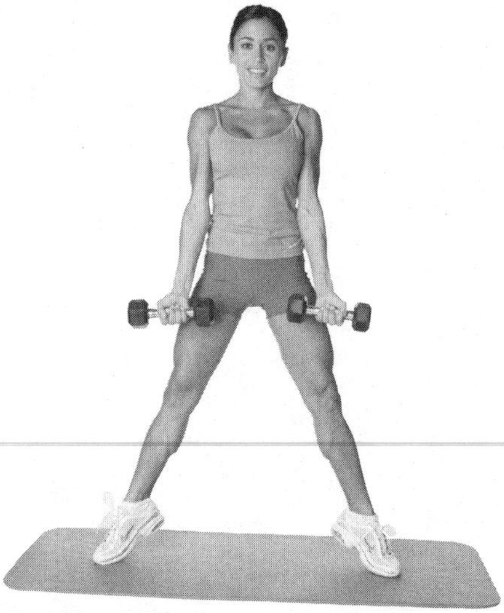

Figure 57

wall sit with front lateral raise (male)

READY: Core, quadriceps, hamstrings, outer thighs, and shoulders

SET: Stand against a wall with a dumbbell in each hand and your palms facing backward. Walk your feet out to 90 degrees and lower your buttocks until you look as if you are sitting in a chair (Figure 58).

Remain in this position throughout the exercise.

GO: Bend your elbows slightly and raise your arms in front of you until the dumbbells reach shoulder level (Figure 59). Lower your arms back to the start position (Figure 58).

modification: You can choose a less-than-seated position to make it easier. You can also do one exercise at a time.

1 set of 20 repetitions

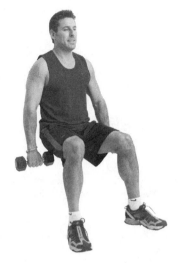

Figure 58

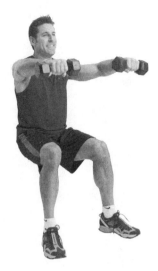

Figure 59

CHAPTER NINE

THE 20 ROUTINE

Throughout the 20 Routine, you will be doing two sets of each exercise. The same parameters apply to the 20 Routine as to the 10 Routine. Make sure to always do some form of light warm-up activity for at least ten minutes prior to doing any form of exercise and also ten minutes of cool down

after exercising. However, because you are completing two sets of each exercise, you may rest in between sets. The optimal rest time is thirty seconds to one minute. You may also rest less than thirty seconds, but try not to rest any longer than one minute. The goal is to work up to needing as little rest as possible. Since there are ten exercises that you will be doing twice each, you may also alternate between exercises if performing two sets back to back is too difficult at the outset. For instance, you may perform one set of the first exercise, then one set of the second exercise repeating the sequence throughout

the entire or partial routine until you are strong enough to do each set of each exercise back to back. Have fun with this routine, as it will be the backbone of your transformation.

For the first six weeks, I recommend you follow the routine for your gender only in the exact order shown here. When you are familiar with your gender's routines, you can customize your workout if you feel a particular exercise better targets an area of the body you wish to focus on. It is important to note that you don't need to customize any of the exercises or routines to meet your goals.

20 ROUTINE

Female	10 Exercises/2 Sets Each	Male	10 Exercises/2 Sets Each
2 sets of 15 reps	Lunge w/Front Kick	2 sets of 10 reps	Mountain Climber w/Push-up
2 sets of 20 reps	Ab Crunch (Legs Up) w/Reverse Crunch	2 sets of 20 reps	Jackknife w/Reverse Crunch(weighted ball)
2 sets of 20 reps	Ab Crunch w/Alternating Leg Extension	2 sets of 20 reps	Ball Chest Press w/Double Triceps Extension
2 sets of 20 reps	Glute Contraction w/Double Triceps Extension	2 sets of 20 reps	Ball Ab Crunch w/Chest Fly
2 sets of 20 reps	Ball Squat w/Shoulder Press	2 sets of 20 reps	Ball Hyperextension w/Rear Lateral Raise
2 sets of 20 reps	Ball Ab Crunch w/Chest Fly	2 sets of 20 reps	Wall Sit w/Biceps Curl and Shoulder Press
2 sets of 20 reps	Ball Glute Contraction w/Double Triceps Kickback	2 sets of 20 reps	Left Lunge Hold w/Double Arm Row and Double Triceps Kickback
2 sets of 20 reps	Left Lunge Hold w/Side Lateral Raise	2 sets of 20 reps	Right Lunge Hold w/Side and Front Lateral Raise
2 sets of 20 reps	Right Lunge Hold w/Biceps Curl	2 sets of 20 reps	Backward Alternating Lunge w/Biceps Curl
2 sets of 20 reps	Squat and Calf Raise w/Front Lateral Raise	2 sets of 20 reps	Squat and Calf Raise w/Front Lateral Raise

lunge with front kick (female)

READY: Core, quadriceps, gluteus maximus, hamstrings, calves, inner thighs, and balance

SET: From a standing position, step forward with your left leg, and drop down into a lunge position, lowering your right knee close to the floor. Keep your back straight at all times. Make sure your left knee is above your left heel every time you come back down into the lunge position. Do not lean forward.

Clench your fists and bring your hands up in front of you into the Pyramid Position (Figure 60), then jab punch with left hand, followed by right cross with right hand.

GO: Raise your right knee into your chest, then extend your right leg from the knee, throwing a snap kick with your toes pointed (Figure 61). Release back down to the start position without putting your foot down until you are back in the lunge position (Figure 60).

modification: Go down into the lunge only as far is comfortable and kick only as high as is comfortable from a balance standpoint.

2 sets of 15 repetitions/kicks on each side

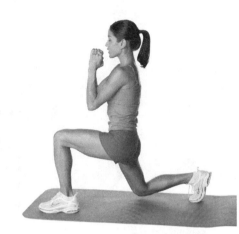

Figure 60

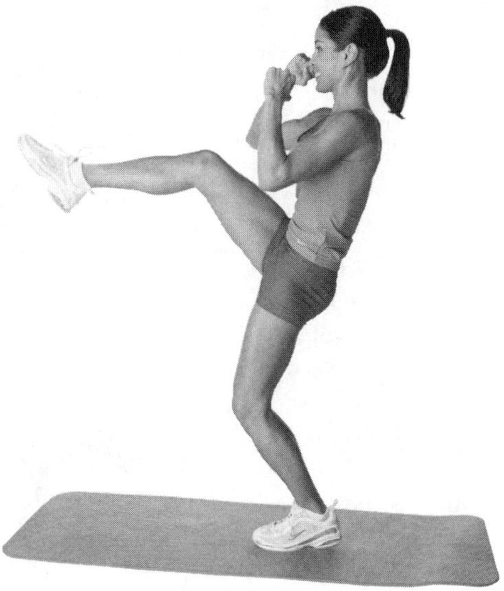

Figure 61

mountain climber with push-up (male)

READY: Core, quadriceps, gluteus maximus, hamstrings, calves, chest, triceps, shoulders, and back

Note: This exercise is performed at a fairly rapid pace, using a four-count.

SET: Start in a plank or push-up position (Figure 62).

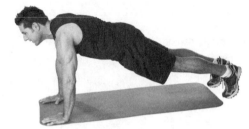

Figure 62

GO: Step your left foot forward toward your left hand (Figure 63). As if you were running, return your left foot to the start position, simultaneously bringing your right foot forward to your right hand (Figure 64). Return your right foot to the start position (Figure 62). From the plank or push-up position, do a push-up with a straight back, pushing back with your heels.

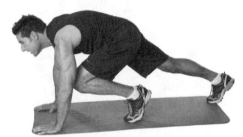

Figure 63

Lower yourself until your chest almost touches the floor (Figure 65).

Push back up into the plank or push-up position (Figure 62) and repeat: left foot forward, right foot forward, push-up.

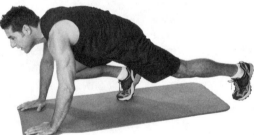

Figure 64

modification: Do one exercise at a time.

2 sets of 10 repetitions

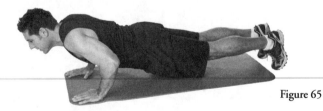

Figure 65

abdominal crunch (legs up) with reverse crunch (female)

READY: Core and upper and lower abdominals

SET: Lie on your back with your knees bent, lift your feet off the floor until your thighs are perpendicular to the floor, cross your ankles, and place your hands behind your head, clasping your fingers together (Figure 66).

GO: Raise your shoulders off the ground in a crunch (Figure 67). Release your upper torso back down to the start position.

Then, using your lower abdominals, lift your buttocks off the ground approximately 2 inches, raising your knees (and feet) upward without swinging your legs too much (Figure 68).

modification: You can lower your legs so that your knees are at a 90-degree angle and raise your knees upward toward your chest. You can also do one exercise at a time.

2 sets of 20 repetitions

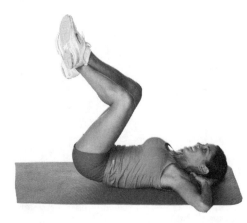

Figure 66

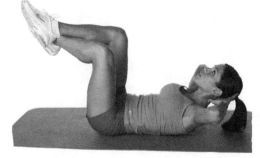

Figure 67

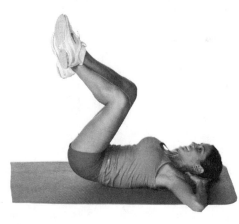

Figure 68

jackknife with reverse crunch (with weighted ball) (male)

READY: core and upper and lower abdominals

SET: Lie on your back with your legs off the floor, your thighs perpendicular to the floor, your knees slightly bent, your ankles crossed. Extend your arms toward your toes with your elbows slightly bent and one hand resting on the other. As you become more advanced, you can hold a weighted ball between your knees or in your hands for added resistance (Figure 69).

GO: Jackknife, reaching up toward your feet and trying to touch your toes (Figure 70).

Release down to the floor. Then, using your lower abdominals, lift your buttocks off the ground approximately 2 inches, raising your knees (and feet) upward without swinging your knees back and forth (Figure 71). Repeat both exercises.

modification: You can do one exercise at a time.

2 sets of 20 repetitions

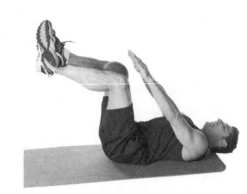

Figure 69

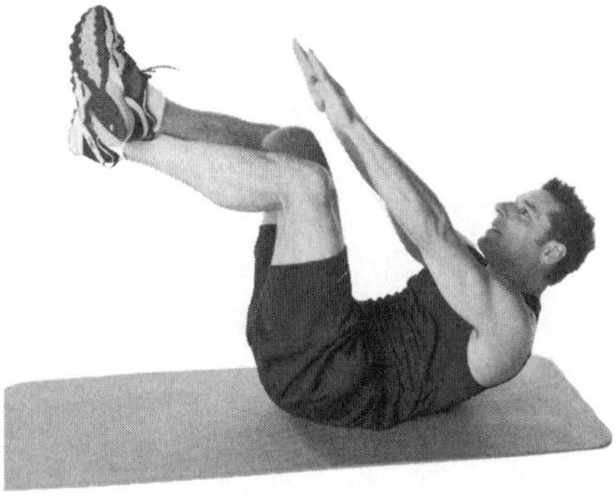

Figure 70

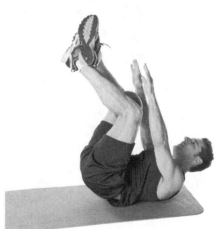

Figure 71

abdominal crunch with alternating leg extension (female)

READY: Core, abdominals, and quadriceps

SET: Put on a pair of 3- to 5-pound ankle weights and lie on the floor. Lie on your back with your knees bent, place your hands behind your head, and clasp your fingers together (Figure 72).

GO: Raise your shoulders off the ground in a crunch.

simultaneously:

Extend your right leg upward into a leg extension, pointing your toes (Figure 73). Release your upper torso back to the start position as you bring your right leg back to the start position.

Repeat with the left leg, alternating with each crunch, until you complete the desired number of repetitions.

modification: You can do one exercise at a time.

2 sets of 20 repetitions

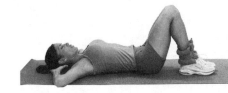

Figure 72

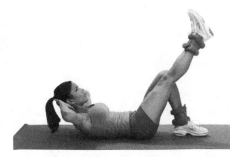

Figure 73

ball chest press with double triceps extension (male)

READY: Core, abdominals, quadriceps, chest, and triceps

SET: Sit on a therapy ball with a dumbbell in each hand. Roll back so that the ball is under your lower to mid back. Position the dumbbells on the same plane as your shoulders. (If you were holding a barbell, it would be lying on top of your collarbone.) Raise your head and tuck in your chin, creating abdominal tension (Figure 74).

GO: Press the dumbbells upward until they almost touch, and hold for a beat (Figure 75). Turn your wrists so the dumbbells are parallel to each other, your palms facing each other (Figure 76). With your arms slightly bent at the elbow, lower the dumbbells toward your shoulders (Figure 77).

Now press the heels of your hands back up (Figure 76). Turn your wrists back into chest press position (Figure 75) and come back down into the start position (Figure 74). Repeat both exercises.

modification: If you have a neck problem or injury, roll the ball out so that your neck is resting on the ball. You can also do one exercise at a time.

2 sets of 20 repetitions

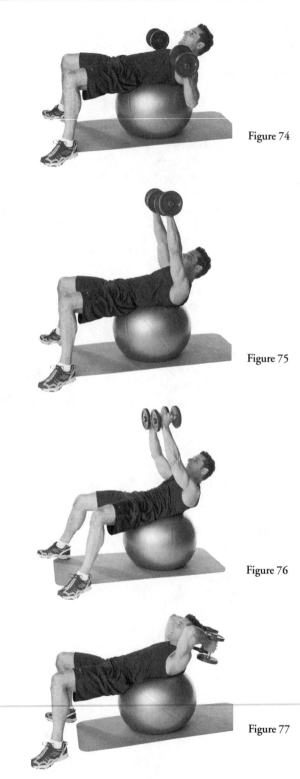

Figure 74

Figure 75

Figure 76

Figure 77

glute contraction with double triceps extension (female)

READY: Core, lower back, gluteus maximus, and triceps

SET: Lie on your back with your knees bent and feet flat on the floor, a dumbbell in each hand. Raise your arms over your torso so they are in alignment with your shoulders, palms facing inward (Figure 78).

Note: You can also place a weighted ball in between your knees to work the inner thighs.

GO: Exhale as you raise your pelvis upward as high as you can, squeezing your buttocks together and contracting your glutes, as you simultaneously lower both dumbbells toward the floor, using your elbow joint as a hinge, keeping both elbows in alignment with your shoulders (Figure 79). Hold for a beat. Lower your pelvis and raise your arms back to the start position. Repeat both exercises.

modification: You can do one exercise at a time.

2 sets of 20 repetitions

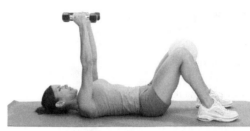

Figure 78

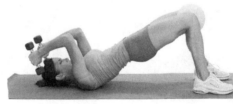

Figure 79

ball abdominal crunch with chest fly (male)

READY: Core, chest, upper and mid abdominals, quadriceps, and triceps

SET: Sit on a therapy ball with a dumbbell in each hand. Roll back so that the ball is under your lower to mid back. Lower the dumbbells until your hands are almost aligned with your shoulders, with your elbows slightly bent, as if you were reaching around a barrel, and tuck your chin into your chest (Figure 80).

GO: Raise your upper torso off the ball into a crunch.

simultaneously:

Push the dumbbells up over your chest, bringing them together and squeezing your chest together (Figure 81). Hold for a beat.

modification: If you have a neck injury or weak abdominals, roll the ball out until your neck is resting on the ball. Do your chest press first and then do your abdominal crunches on the ball separately until you are strong enough to do both together (Figures 82 and 83).

2 sets of 20 repetitions

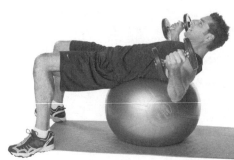

Figure 80

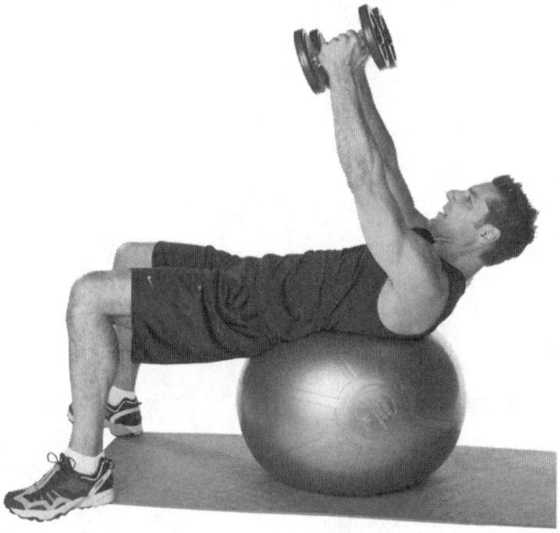

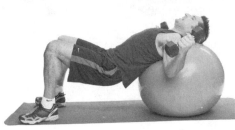

Figure 81

Figure 82

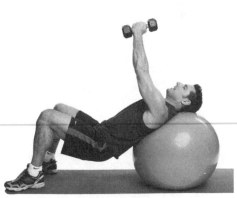

Figure 83

ball squat with shoulder press (female)

READY: Core, quadriceps, hamstrings, gluteus maximus, outer thighs, lower back, and shoulders

SET: With a dumbbell in each hand, stand with the therapy ball between you and a wall, resting in the small of your lower back, your feet slightly more than shoulder width apart, your toes turned out slightly. Bring your arms into a "goalpost" position above your head with your elbows in alignment with your shoulders and your palms facing forward (Figure 84).

GO: Exhaling, bend at your knees, lowering your torso until you look as if you are sitting in a chair, simultaneously pressing the dumbbells upward until your elbows almost lock and your hands are directly above your shoulders (Figure 85). Return to the start position. Repeat.

modification: You can do one exercise at a time.

2 sets of 20 repetitions

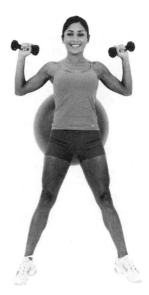

Figure 84

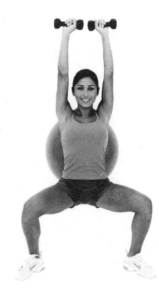

Figure 85

ball hyperextension with rear lateral raise (male)

READY: Core, back, lower back, calves, gluteus maximus, and shoulders

SET: Lie on your stomach on a therapy ball with a dumbbell in each hand. Position the ball just under your diaphragm and place your feet against a wall or a stationary object. Drape your arms over the front of the ball, your elbows bent, your palms facing each other (Figure 86).

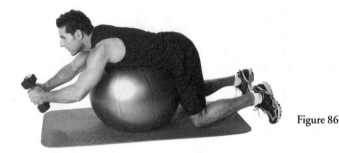

Figure 86

GO: Raise your torso and straighten your body until it is in one straight line from your head to your feet.

simultaneously:

As you arch up, lift your slightly bent arms back and outward, squeezing your shoulder blades together (Figure 87). Hold for a beat. Release back down into the start position.

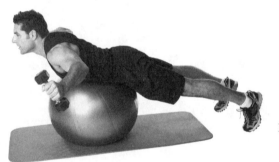

Figure 87

modification: You can do one exercise at a time. If you have an extremely weak lower back, you can begin with hyperextensions lying on your stomach, on a floor mat. Initially raise only your outstretched arms; then, after a while, raise your outstretched arms and legs simultaneously with your ankles crossed. When you feel strong enough, move on to the ball.

2 sets of 20 repetitions

ball abdominal crunch with chest fly (female)

READY: Core, upper and mid abdominals, chest, quadriceps, and triceps

SET: Sit on a therapy ball with a dumbbell in each hand. Roll back so that the ball is under your lower to mid back. Raise your head, and tuck your chin into your chest.

Lower the dumbbells until your hands are almost in alignment with your shoulders, your elbows slightly bent as if you were reaching around a barrel (Figure 88).

GO: Raise your arms directly over your chest until the dumbbells come together, simultaneously raising your torso into an abdominal crunch (Figure 89). Hold for a beat. Release your torso and arms back to the start position.

modification: You can do one exercise at a time. If you have a neck injury or weak abdominals, roll the ball out until your neck is resting on the ball (Figure 88). Do your chest presses first and then do your abdominal crunches on the ball separately until you are strong enough to do both together.

2 sets of 20 repetitions

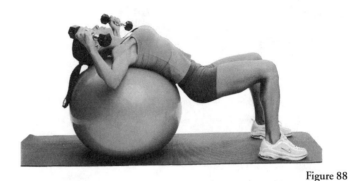

Figure 88

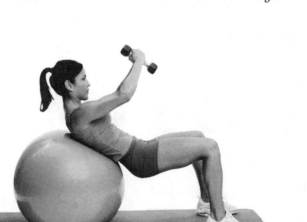

Figure 89

wall sit with biceps curl and shoulder press (male)

READY: core, quadriceps, shoulders, and biceps

SET: Stand against a wall with a dumbbell in each hand, your palms facing inward. Walk your feet out and lower your buttocks until you look as if you are sitting in a chair with your feet directly under your knees (Figure 90).

Remain in this position throughout the exercise.

GO: Raise the dumbbells to your chest in a curling motion, twisting your wrists slightly so the backs of your hands are directed toward each other, keeping your elbows tight into your rib cage until you get to the top of the movement (Figure 91). Then bring your arms upward into the goalpost position with your palms facing forward (Figure 92). Raise the dumbbells straight overhead until your elbows almost lock (Figure 93). Lower your arms back to start position (Figure 90).

modification: You can choose a less-than-seated position to make the exercise easier.

2 sets of 20 repetitions

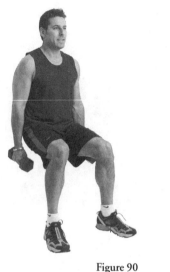

Figure 90

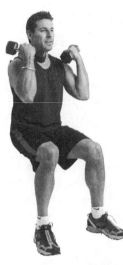

Figure 91

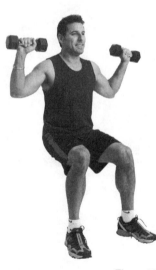

Figure 92

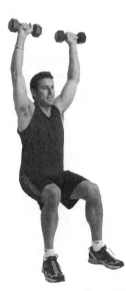

Figure 93

ball glute contraction with double triceps kickback (female)

READY: Core, lower back, back, gluteus maximus, and triceps

SET: Lie on your stomach on a therapy ball with a dumbbell in each hand and your feet against a wall or a stationary object. Drape your torso over the ball. Bring your elbows up tight into your rib cage with your elbows raised as high as possible (Figure 94).

GO: Roll out onto the ball and arch your back so that your body is in a straight line, squeezing your buttocks together.

simultaneously:

Extend your arms backward from the elbow as far as you can (Figure 95). Hold for a beat. Then release your torso and arms back down to the start position.

modification: You can do one exercise at a time, resting your hands behind your back on the glute contraction and resting your torso on the ball for the kickbacks.

2 sets of 20 repetitions

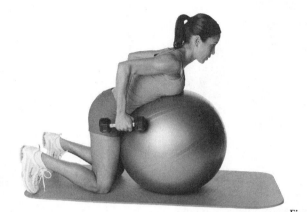

Figure 94

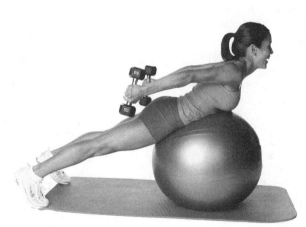

Figure 95

left lunge hold with double arm row and double triceps kickback (male)

READY: Core, quadriceps, hamstrings, gluteus maximus, calves, inner thighs, back, triceps, and balance

SET: Stand with a dumbbell in each hand. Step forward with your left foot, dropping your right knee close to the floor and keeping your left knee directly above your left heel. Lean forward so that your chest is almost resting on your left thigh, arching your back slightly. Your arms are extended below you, the dumbbells are close to the floor, and your palms are facing backward (Figure 96).

Remain in this position throughout the exercise.

GO: In a rowing motion, bring the dumbbells up until they are level with your rib cage, twisting your wrists slowly as you come up so that at the end of the movement the dumbbells are parallel with your body. Keep your elbows as high as you can and tightly into your rib cage (Figure 97).

Using your elbow joint as a hinge, extend your arms backward, leading with the heels of your hands, until your arms are fully extended (Figure 98). Hold for a beat, unlock your elbows, and release your arms back down toward the ground into the start

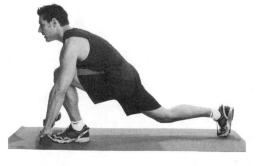

Figure 96

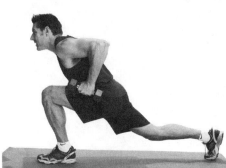

Figure 97

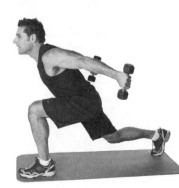

Figure 98

position (Figure 96). Repeat both exercises.

modification: You can do one exercise at a time.

2 sets of 20 repetitions

left lunge hold with side lateral raise (female)

READY: Core, quadriceps, hamstrings, gluteus maximus, calves, inner thighs, shoulders, and balance

SET: Stand with a dumbbell in each hand, your arms by your sides, your palms facing inward. Step forward with your left foot, dropping your right knee close to the floor and keeping your left knee directly above your left heel, your back straight (Figure 99).

Remain in this position throughout the exercise.

GO: With slightly bent arms, lift the dumbbells out to the sides until your hands reach eye level (Figure 100). Lower the dumbbells back to the start position (Figure 99).

modification: You can do one exercise at a time.

2 sets of 20 repetitions

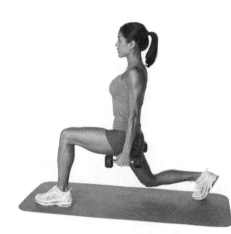

Figure 99

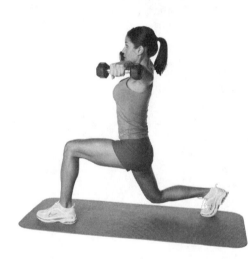

Figure 100

right lunge hold with side and front lateral raise (male)

READY: Core, quadriceps, hamstrings, gluteus maximus, calves, inner thighs, back, shoulders, and balance

SET: Stand with a dumbbell in each hand, your palms facing inward, your elbows slightly bent. Step out with your right foot into a lunge position with your right knee directly above your right heel, your back straight (Figure 101).

Remain in this position throughout the exercise.

GO: Lift the dumbbells out to the sides up to eye level (Figure 102). Lower your arms and twist your wrists so your palms are facing backward. Raise your arms forward to shoulder level (Figure 103). Lower them back to the start position (Figure 101). Repeat both exercises.

modification: You can do one exercise at a time.

2 sets of 20 repetitions

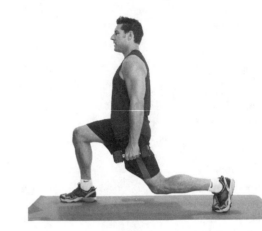

Figure 101

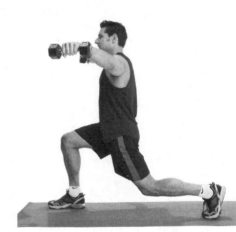

Figure 102

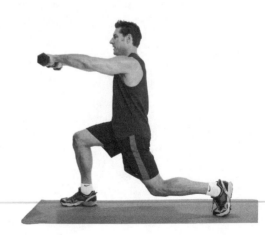

Figure 103

right lunge hold with biceps curl (female)

READY: Core, quadriceps, hamstrings, gluteus maximus, calves, inner thighs, biceps, and balance

SET: Stand with a dumbbell in each hand, palms facing forward, your arms by your side. Step out with your right foot into a lunge position, your right knee directly above your right foot, your back straight (Figure 104).

Remain in position throughout the exercise.

GO: Curl your hands up toward your shoulders, keeping your elbows tight against your rib cage, and at the top of the movement, twist your wrists slightly so the backs of your hands are directed toward each other (Figure 105). Lower your arms (Figure 104).

modification: You can do one exercise at a time.

2 sets of 20 repetitions

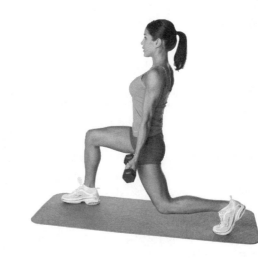

Figure 104

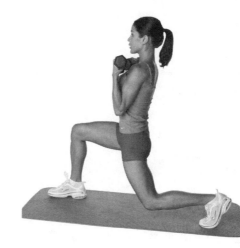

Figure 105

backward alternating lunge with biceps curl (male)

READY: Core, quadriceps, hamstrings, gluteus maximus, calves, inner thighs, biceps, and balance

SET: Stand with a dumbbell in each hand, your arms by your sides (Figure 106).

GO: Step backward with your right foot, going down into a lunge position, your left knee directly above your left heel, your back straight.

simultaneously:

Curl your hands up toward your shoulders, keeping your elbows tight against your rib cage, and at the top of the movement, twist your wrists slightly so the backs of your hands are directed toward each other (Figure 107).

Then step forward with your right foot as you stand back up and lower your arms back to the start position (Figure 106). Alternate legs on every repetition.

modification: You can do one exercise at a time.

2 sets of 20 repetitions

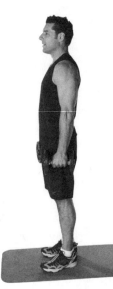

Figure 106

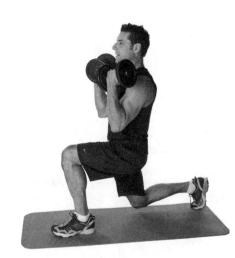

Figure 107

squat and calf raise with front lateral raise (female)

READY: Core, quadriceps, hamstrings, gluteus maximus, outer thighs, calves, lower back, and shoulders

SET: Stand with a dumbbell in each hand, your palms facing backward, your feet slightly more than shoulder width apart, your toes turned out slightly (Figure 108).

GO: Arch your back slightly, keeping your torso over your pelvis. Then lower yourself as if you were sitting in a chair, going down as far as is comfortable.

simultaneously:

Raise your slightly bent arms up to just eye level (Figure 109). Then slowly lower your arms as you come back up to the standing position (Figure 108).

Jut your hips forward slightly to get a glute contraction. Rise up onto your toes in an explosive movement, contracting your calves (Figure 110). Hold for a beat, then release back to the floor.

2 sets of 20 repetitions

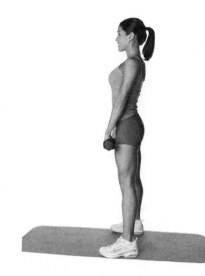

Figure 108

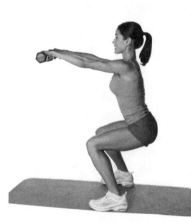

Figure 109

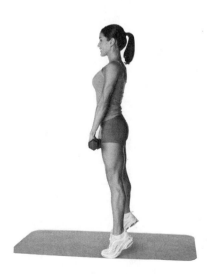

Figure 110

squat and calf raise with front lateral raise (male)

READY: Core, quadriceps, hamstrings, gluteus maximus, outer thighs, calves, lower back, and shoulders

SET: Stand with a dumbbell in each hand, your palms facing backward, your feet slightly more than shoulder width apart, your toes turned out slightly (Figure 111).

GO: Arch your back slightly, keeping your torso over your pelvis. Then lower yourself as if you were sitting in a chair, going down as far as is comfortable.

simultaneously:

With your arms slightly bent, raise the dumbbells just above shoulder level (Figure 112). Then slowly lower your arms as you come back up to the start position (Figure 113).

Jut your hips forward slightly to get a glute contraction and rise up onto your toes in an explosive movement, contracting your calves. Hold for a beat (Figure 114). Then release back to the floor.

modification: You can do one exercise at a time.

2 sets of 20 repetitions

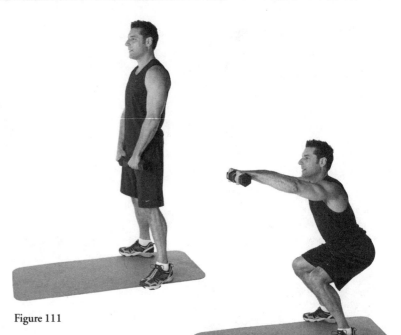

Figure 111

Figure 112

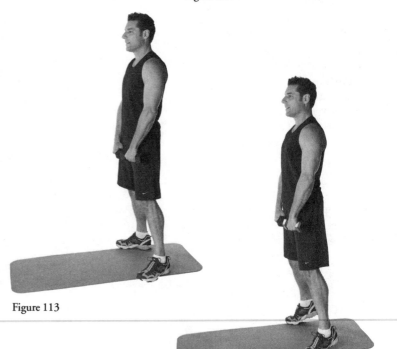

Figure 113

Figure 114

CHAPTER TEN

THE 30 ROUTINE

Throughout the 30 Routine, you will be doing three sets of each exercise. The same parameters apply to the 30 Routine as to the 10 and 20 Routines. Make sure to always do some form of light warm-up activity for at least ten minutes prior to doing any form of exercise and also ten minutes of cool down after exercising. However, because you are now completing three sets of each exercise, you may need more rest in between sets. Remember, the optimal rest time is thirty seconds to one minute. You may rest less than thirty seconds, but try not to rest longer than one minute. Work up to this if you have to. Since there are ten exercises that you will be doing three times each, you may also alternate between exercises if performing three sets of one exercise back to back is too difficult at the outset. For instance, you may perform one set of the first exercise, then one set of the second exercise, repeating the sequence throughout the entire or partial routine, depending upon your strengths and weaknesses. Do this for the entire routine until you are strong enough to do each set of each ex- ercise back to back. This is probably one of the most challenging exercise routines you will ever do, so be patient at first and don't beat yourself up if it takes longer than you feel it should or if you cannot complete the entire routine. In time you will be able to do the entire routine in the right time.

For the first six weeks, I recommend you follow the routine for your gender only in the exact order shown here. When you are familiar with your gender's routines, you can customize your workout if you feel a particular exercise better targets an area of the body you wish to focus on. It is important to note that you don't need to customize any of the exercises or routines to meet your goals.

30 ROUTINE

Female	10 Exercises/3 Sets Each	Male	10 Exercises/3 Sets Each
3 sets of 15 reps	One-Two Punch w/Lunge Kick (hand weights optional)	3 sets of 15 reps	Push-up w/Alternating Dumbbell Row
3 sets of 20 reps	Ab Crunch w/Alternating Leg Extension and Inner Thigh Squeeze (ankle weights, weighted ball)	3 sets of 20 reps	Side Oblique Crunch w/Rear Lateral Raise
		3 sets of 20 reps	Weighted Crunch w/Reverse Crunch (dumbbell or weighted ball)
3 sets of 20 reps	Side Crunch w/Side Leg Raise (ankle weights)	3 sets of 20 reps	Ball Chest Press w/Chest Fly
3 sets of 20 reps	Standing Glute Kickback w/Opposite Triceps Kickback (ankle weights)	3 sets of 20 reps	Alternating Lunge w/Shoulder Press
		3 sets of 20 reps	Right Lunge Hold w/Side Lateral Raise
3 sets of 20 reps	Ball Chest Press w/Chest Fly	3 sets of 20 reps	Left Lunge Hold w/Double Triceps Extension
3 sets of 20 reps	Alternating Step-up Biceps Curl w/Shoulder Press	3 sets of 20 reps	Right Closed T-stance w/Front Lateral Raise
3 sets of 20 reps	Right Closed T-stance w/Double Triceps Extension	3 sets of 20 reps	Left Closed T-stance w/Biceps Curl
3 sets of 20 reps	Left Closed T-stance w/Front Lateral Raise	3 sets of 20 reps	Squat and Calf Raise w/Double Triceps Kickback
3 sets of 20 reps	Right Warrior Pose w/Side Lateral Raise		
3 sets of 20 reps	Left Lunge Hold w/Double Row and Double Triceps Kickback		

one-two punch with lunge kick (female)

READY: Core, quadriceps, gluteus maximus, hamstrings, calves, inner thighs, biceps, back, shoulders, triceps, and balance

SET: Stand with a 3- to 5-pound dumbbell in each hand. Step forward with your left leg and drop down into a lunge position, lowering your right knee close to the floor and keeping your back straight at all times. Do not lean forward. Make sure your left knee is directly above your left heel every time you come back down onto the lunge position. Your arms are in the Pyramid Position with your hands clenched (Figure 115).

GO: Punch with your left arm and then with your right arm (Figures 116 and 117). At the end of the second punch, immediately raise your right knee up toward your chest, then extend the right leg from the knee and throw a snap kick with your toe pointed (Figure 118). Release back down to the start position without putting your foot down until you are back in the lunge position (Figure 115).

modification: Go down into the lunge only as far as is comfortable from a strength perspective and kick only as high as is comfortable from a balance perspective. You can also do the exercise without the dumbbells or do one exercise at a time.

3 sets of 15 repetitions/kicks on both sides

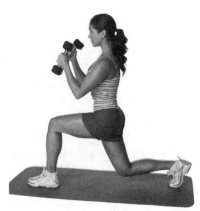

Figure 115

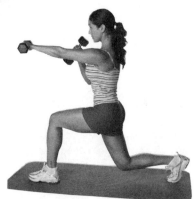

Figure 116

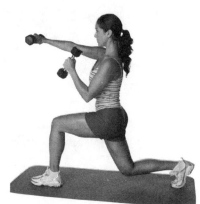

Figure 117

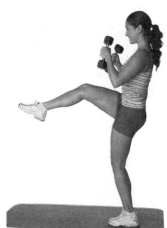

Figure 118

push-up with alternating dumbbell row (male)

READY: Core, back, lower back, chest, triceps, and balance

SET: Place a pair of dumbbells on the floor in front of you. Move into a push-up position with your hands on the dumbbells. With a straight lower back, push back on your heels (Figure 119).

GO: Lower yourself until your chest almost touches the dumbbells (Figure 120).

simultaneously:

Then, as you push back up, lift your left arm off the ground and twist your wrist inward in a one-arm rowing motion, keeping the dumbbell close to your rib cage (Figure 121). Lower your torso and release your left arm back to the start position (Figure 119). Repeat on the other side, alternating arms on every repetition.

modification: Do only one exercise at a time. Do the alternating dumbbell row with one leg and one hand on a chair, arm dangling. Do the row to completion on one side and then switch to the other side.

3 sets of 15 repetitions

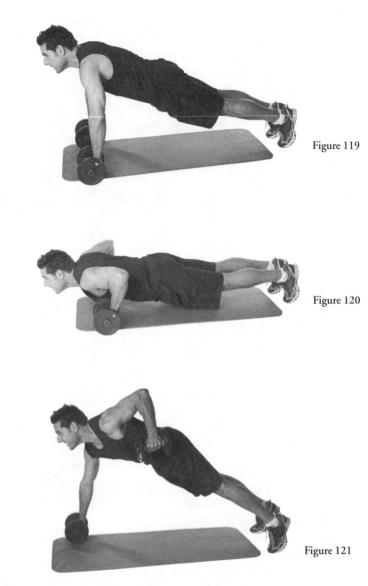

Figure 119

Figure 120

Figure 121

abdominal crunch with alternating leg extension and inner thigh squeeze (with ankle weights and weighted ball) (female)

READY: Core, abdominals, quadriceps, and inner thighs

SET: Put on a pair of 3- to 5-pound ankle weights and lie on your back. Keep your knees bent, your feet flat on the floor, and put a weighted ball between your inner thighs around the knee area. Place your hands behind your head, interlocking your fingers (Figure 122).

GO: Squeeze the weighted ball tightly with your inner thighs as you raise your shoulders off the ground into a crunch while simultaneously extending your left foot, keeping your foot flexed, into a full extension (Figure 123). Release back down and repeat with the right leg, alternating legs until you complete the desired number of repetitions.

modification: Do the exercise without the weighted ball between your thighs (Figures 124 and 125).

3 sets of 20 repetitions

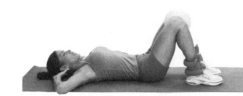

Figure 122

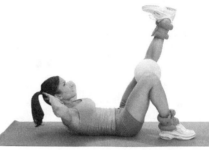

Figure 123

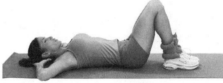

Figure 124

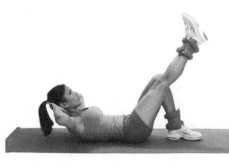

Figure 125

side oblique crunch with rear lateral raise (male)

READY: Core, abdominals, obliques, shoulders, and balance

SET: Lie on your right side with a dumbbell in your left hand and your left arm outstretched in front of your torso. Place your right arm across the front of the mat so that you can support your weight on that arm. Bring your bent knees up toward your chest (Figure 126).

Note: The higher up you bring your bent knees in to your chest, the harder you will work your obliques.

GO: Raise your right hip as high as you can, digging the edges of both feet into the mat for support (so you don't slide downward) and rolling your hip slightly forward at the top of the movement.

simultaneously:

Raise your slightly bent arm upward about 2 to 3 feet (Figure 127). Lower yourself and repeat the exercise. Then switch to the other side.

modification: This is an extremely difficult exercise. You can do one exercise at a time or do the exercise on page 102 (George's Oblique) for your obliques and do the rear lateral raise separately by standing with bent knees and an arched back, your arms outstretched in front of you, then bringing your arms back, squeezing your shoulder blades together, and finally releasing your arms back to the front.

3 sets of 20 repetitions

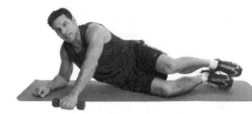

Figure 126

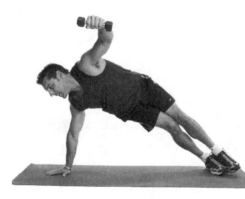

Figure 127

side crunch with side leg raise (with ankle weights) (female)

READY: Abdominals, obliques, outer thighs, and balance

SET: With ankle weights on, lie on your back and twist your lower body onto your left side, keeping your upper torso flat on the mat with your right hand behind your head. Bend your left leg slightly toward your chest, tucked under your right leg. Extend your right leg fully. Drape your left arm across your waist.

Note: Place your arm on the floor beside your torso for balance support. Your right hand should be behind your head supporting it. (Figure 128).

GO: Twist your torso as you bring your right elbow up toward your left knee.

simultaneously:

Raise your right leg 2 to 3 feet, pushing out with the heel (Figure 129). Release back down and repeat the exercise for the full set of repetitions. Then switch to the other side.

modification: You can do one exercise at a time.

3 sets of 20 repetitions on both sides

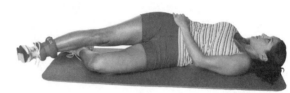

Figure 128

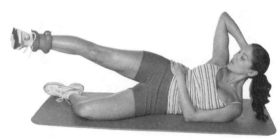

Figure 129

weighted crunch with reverse crunch (with dumbbell or weighted ball) (male)

READY: Core, abdominals, obliques, and shoulders

SET: Lie on your back with your legs bent, feet flat on the floor. Either hold a weighted (medicine) ball in your outstretched hands or hold the sides of a dumbbell.

With your ankles crossed and a weighted ball between your thighs, bring your legs up until your thighs are perpendicular to the ground. Your arms should be almost fully extended above your chest with your elbows slightly bent (Figure 130).

GO: Lift your shoulders off the floor into a crunch, pushing the weighted ball or dumbbell straight up as high as you can (Figure 131). Release and come back down (Figure 130). Then, using your lower abdominals, lift your buttocks off the ground approximately 2 inches, raising your knees (and feet) upward without swinging your knees back and forth (Figure 132). Repeat until you complete the desired number of repetitions.

modification: You can do one exercise at a time or do the crunch without a dumbbell.

3 sets of 20 repetitions

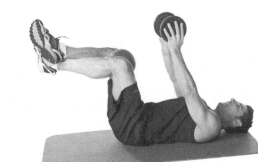

Figure 130

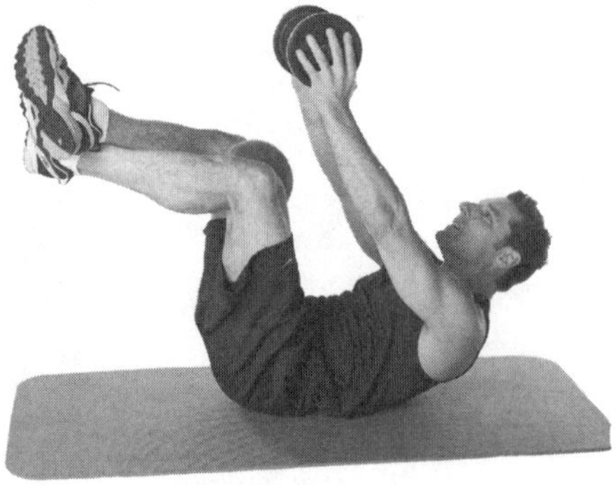

Figure 131

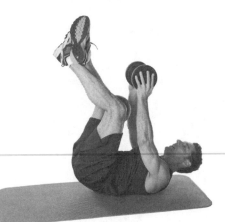

Figure 132

standing glute kickback with opposite triceps kickback (with ankle weights) (female)

READY: Hips, quadriceps, hamstrings, gluteus maximus, lower back, triceps, and balance

SET: Stand facing a chair, wall, or bar with 3- to 5-pound ankle weights on and a dumbbell in your right hand. Hold on to the chair, wall, or bar with your left hand and lean forward. Bring your right elbow up as high as you can, keeping your arm close to your rib cage, as you bring your left knee up toward your chest (Figure 133).

GO: Extend your left leg backward, pushing back with the heel and keeping your entire torso in one plane and in alignment.

simultaneously:

Extend your right arm backward, keeping your elbow up high (Figure 134). Release and return to the start position (Figure 133). Complete one set of reps, then switch to the other side, alternating sides as you move through the desired number of sets.

modification: You can do one exercise at a time. You can also do the exercise without ankle weights.

3 sets of 20 repetitions on both sides

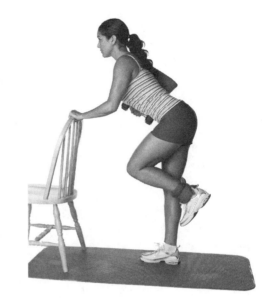

Figure 133

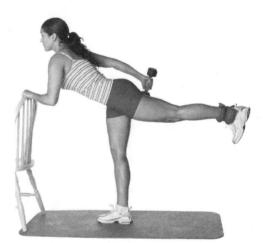

Figure 134

ball chest press with chest fly (male)

READY: Chest, lower back, abdominals, quadriceps, and triceps

SET: Sit on a therapy ball, with a dumbbell in each hand. Roll back so that the ball is underneath your mid to lower back. Position the dumbbells on the same plane as your shoulders. (If you were holding a barbell, it would be lying on top of your collarbone.) Raise your head slightly and tuck in your chin, creating abdominal tension (Figure 135).

GO: Press the dumbbells upward until your arms are almost fully extended and hold for a beat as you squeeze your chest muscles together (Figure 136). Then twist your wrists so the dumbbells are parallel with your body (Figure 137).

Lower your slightly bent arms out to the sides, feeling the stretch across your chest on the way down, until the dumbbells are level with your shoulders (Figure 138). Press the dumbbells up again as though you were reaching around a barrel, bringing them together as you extend your arms (Figure 137). Hold for a beat. Twist your wrists back and lower your arms into the start position (Figure 135).

modification: If you have a neck injury or weak abdominals, roll out on the ball until your neck is resting on the ball and use lighter hand weights (see p. 103).

3 sets of 20 repetitions

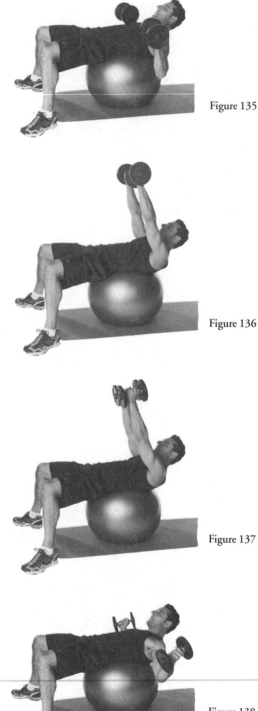

Figure 135

Figure 136

Figure 137

Figure 138

ball chest press with chest fly (female)

READY: Chest, lower back, abdominals, quadriceps, and triceps

SET: Sit on a therapy ball with a dumbbell in each hand. Roll back so that the ball is underneath your mid to lower back. Position the dumbbells on the same plane as your shoulders. (If you were holding a barbell, it would be lying on top of your collarbone.) Raise your head slightly and tuck in your chin, creating abdominal tension (Figure 139).

GO: Press the dumbbells upward until your arms are almost fully extended and hold for a beat as you squeeze your chest muscles together (Figure 140). Then twist your wrists so the dumbbells are parallel with your body (Figure 141).

Lower your slightly bent arms out to the sides, feeling the stretch across your chest on the way down, until the dumbbells are level with your shoulders (Figure 142). Press the dumbbells up again as though you were reaching around a barrel, bringing them together as you extend your arms. (Figure 141). Hold for a beat. Twist your wrists back and lower your arms into the start position (Figure 139).

modification: If you have a neck injury or weak abdominals, roll out on the ball until your neck is resting on the ball (see p. 103).

3 sets of 20 repetitions

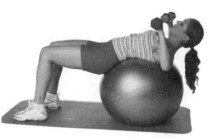

Figure 139

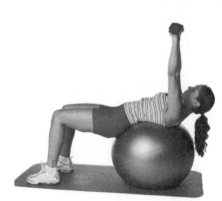

Figure 140

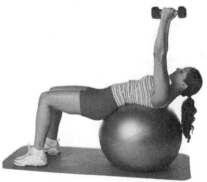

Figure 141

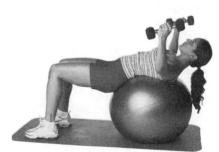

Figure 142

alternating lunge with shoulder press (male)

READY: Core, quadriceps, gluteus maximus, hamstrings, calves, inner thighs, shoulders, and balance

SET: Stand with a dumbbell in each hand. Position the dumbbells in the goalpost or shoulder press position (Figure 143).

GO: Step out with your left foot and come down into a lunge, keeping your left knee directly over your left heel and your back straight.

simultaneously:

Press the dumbbells upward until your arms are fully extended (Figure 144). Step back into standing position as you lower your arms back into the goalpost position. Repeat, stepping out with your right foot. Alternate legs until you complete the repetitions.

modification: Go down into the lunge only as far as is comfortable. In time your legs will be strong enough to go all the way down.

3 sets of 20 repetitions

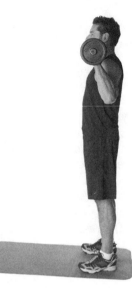

Figure 143

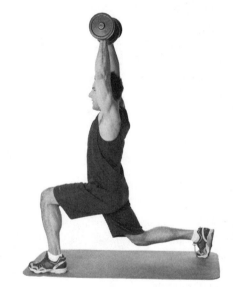

Figure 144

alternating step-up biceps curl with shoulder press (female)

READY: Core, quadriceps, hamstrings, gluteus maximus, biceps, shoulders, triceps, and balance

This exercise can be performed using stairs, a step, or a sturdy chair, box, or bench. You just need to make sure the platform is big enough to stand on with both feet and sturdy enough to support your entire body weight. You also want to make sure the platform is not too high. You will know if it is too high if you have to lean forward when stepping.

SET: Stand with a dumbbell in each hand, facing the platform, palms facing inward (Figure 145).

GO: Step up onto the platform with your right leg (Figure 146).

simultaneously:

Do a biceps curl, keeping your elbows in tight to your rib cage (Figure 146), and at the top of the movement, twist your wrists slightly so the backs of your hands are directed toward each other. As your left foot comes up on top of the platform so you are once again standing, move your arms into the goalpost or shoulder press position (Figure 147). Press the dumbbells upward until your arms are fully extended (Figure 148). Release the dumbbells back to your sides as you step off the platform (Figure 145). Repeat the exercise, alternating legs. Begin each set with the opposite leg from the previous set.

3 sets of 20 repetitions

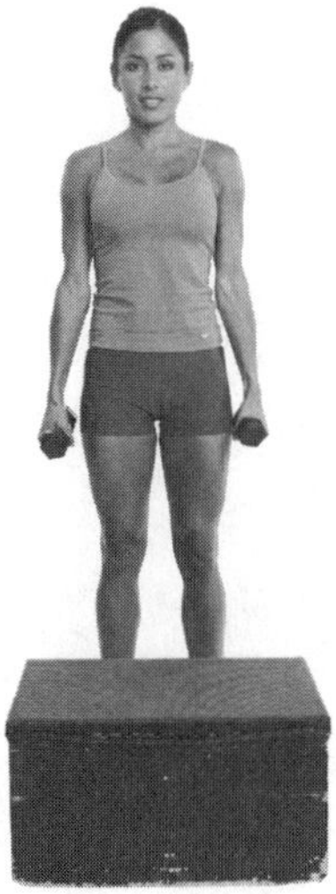

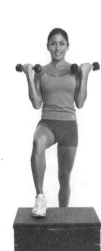

Figure 145

Figure 146

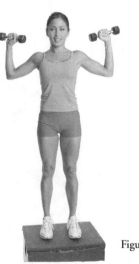

Figure 147

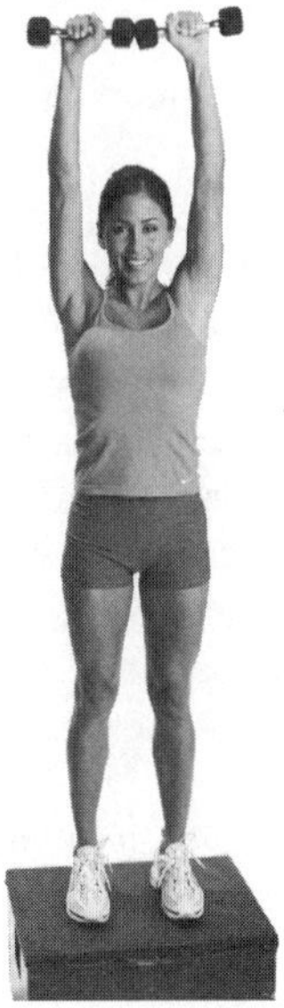

Figure 148

right lunge hold with side lateral raise (male)

READY: Core, quadriceps, hamstrings, gluteus maximus, calves, inner thighs, back, shoulders, and balance

SET: Stand with a dumbbell in each hand, your palms facing inward, your elbows slightly bent (Figure 149). Step out with your right foot into a lunge position with your right knee directly above your right heel, your back straight (Figure 150).

Remain in this position throughout the exercise.

GO: Lift the dumbbells out to the sides up to eye level (Figure 151). Lower your arms and twist your wrists so your palms are facing backward. Raise your arms forward to shoulder level. Lower them, then twist your wrists again back to the start position (Figure 149). Repeat both exercises.

modification: You can do one exercise at a time.

3 sets of 20 repetitions

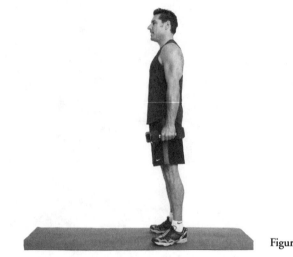

Figure 149

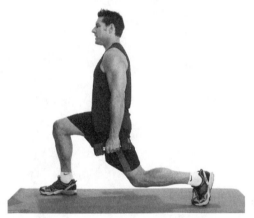

Figure 150

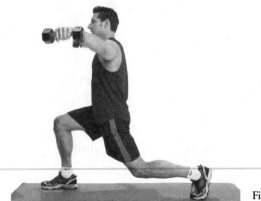

Figure 151

right closed t-stance with double triceps extension (female)

READY: Quadriceps, hamstrings, calves, gluteus maximus, lower back, shoulders, and balance

SET: Stand with a dumbbell in each hand. Bring your right foot behind your left leg and lower yourself down as far as is comfortable, almost in a curtsey, placing the ball of your right foot outside your left foot as far as is comfortable. Bend your left knee and drop down as far as you can, keeping your hips and torso square to the front as much as possible.

Remain in this position throughout the entire exercise.

Raise your arms over your head so that your elbows are facing forward and are close to your ears (Figure 152).

GO: Release your arms from the elbow hinge and lower the dumbbells down to your shoulders (Figure 153) and then back up to start, and repeat the exercise until you complete the desired repetitions.

modification: You can do one exercise at a time. Only go down as far as is comfortable.

3 sets of 20 repetitions

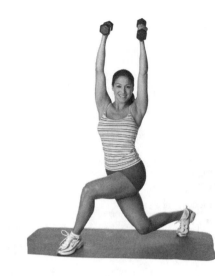

Figure 152

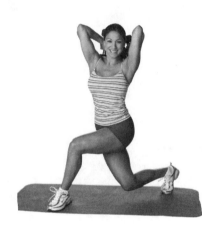

Figure 153

left lunge hold with double triceps extension (male)

READY: Core, quadriceps, gluteus maximus, hamstrings, calves, inner thighs, triceps, and balance

SET: Stand with a dumbbell in each hand, your palms facing inward. Step forward with your left foot. Lower your right knee close to the floor. Make sure your right knee is directly above your right heel and at a 90-degree angle.

Remain in this position throughout the entire exercise.

GO: Raise your arms over your head so that your elbows are facing forward and are close to your ears (Figure 154). Release your arms from the elbow hinge and lower the dumbbells to your shoulders (Figure 155). Raise your arms back to the start position.

modification: You can do one exercise at a time, or don't go all the way down in the lunge.

3 sets of 20 repetitions

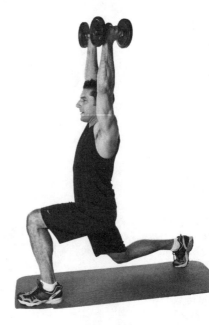

Figure 154

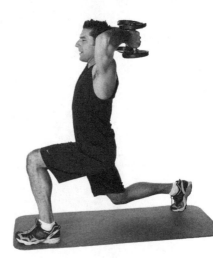

Figure 155

left closed t-stance with front lateral raise (female)

READY: Quadriceps, hamstrings, calves, gluteus maximus, lower back, shoulders, and balance

SET: Stand with a dumbbell in each hand, your palms facing backward. Bring your left foot behind your right leg and lower yourself down as far as is comfortable, almost in a curtsey, positioning the ball of your left foot outside your right foot as far as is comfortable and keeping your hips and torso as square to the front as possible (Figure 156).

Remain in this position throughout the exercise.

GO: With your arms slightly bent, raise the dumbbells in front of you until they reach eye level (Figures 157 and 158). Lower them slightly, and repeat until you complete the desired number of repetitions.

3 sets of 20 repetitions

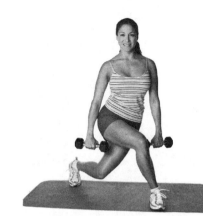

Figure 156

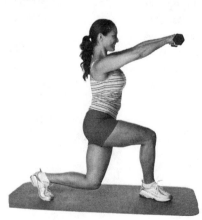

Figure 157

Figure 158

157

right closed t-stance with front lateral raise (male)

READY: Quadriceps, hamstrings, calves, gluteus maximus, lower back, shoulders, and balance

SET: Stand with a dumbbell in each hand, your palms facing inward (Figure 159). Bring your right foot behind your left leg and lower yourself down as far as is comfortable, almost in a curtsey, positioning the ball of your right foot outside your left foot as far as is comfortable and keeping your hips and torso as square to the front as possible (Figure 160).

Remain in this position throughout the exercise.

GO: With your arms slightly bent, raise the dumbbells in front of you until they reach almost eye level (Figures 161 and 162). Lower them and repeat until you complete the desired number of repetitions. Repeat the exercise with your left foot behind your right leg.

modification: Don't go down in the stance too far.

3 sets of 20 repetitions

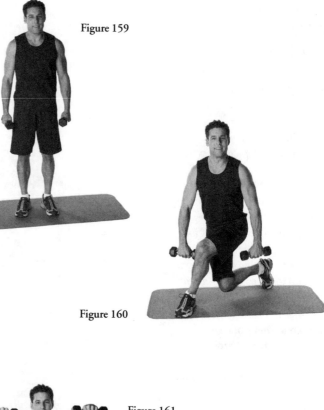

Figure 159

Figure 160

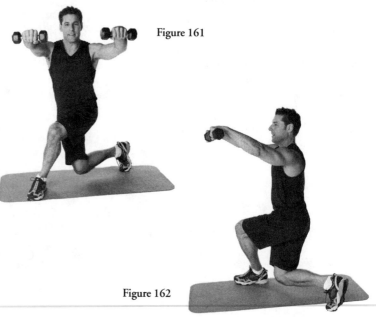

Figure 161

Figure 162

right warrior pose with side lateral raise (female)

READY: Core, quadriceps, gluteus maximus, hamstrings, calves, inner thighs, shoulders, and balance

SET: Stand with a dumbbell in each hand hanging in front of you, palms facing inward. Step forward with your left foot and pivot your right foot outward until it is perpendicular to your left foot. Your left heel should be in alignment with your right heel. Rotate your torso so that you face in the same direction as your right foot. Bend your left knee and drop down as far as you can, preferably so that your left knee is at a 90-degree angle (Figure 163). Focus on your breathing.

Remain in this position throughout the exercise.

GO: With your arms in front of your torso and your elbows slightly bent, sweep your arms out to the sides until the dumbbells reach almost eye level (Figure 164). Lower the dumbbells and repeat the exercise.

modification: Only go down as far as feels comfortable.

3 sets of 20 repetitions

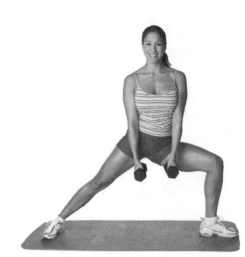

Figure 163

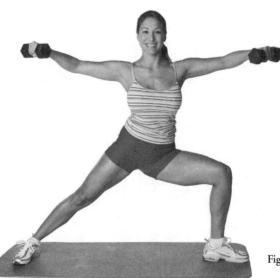

Figure 164

left closed t-stance with biceps curl (male)

READY: Quadriceps, hamstrings, calves, gluteus maximus, lower back, biceps, and balance

SET: Stand with dumbbells in each hand, palms facing forward. Bring your left foot behind your right leg and lower yourself down as far as is comfortable, almost in a curtsey, positioning the ball of your left foot outside your right foot and keeping your torso as square to the front as possible (Figure 165).

Remain in this position throughout the exercise.

GO: Raise your arms upward in a curling motion, keeping your elbows in tight to your rib cage, and at the top of the movement, twist your wrists slightly so the backs of your hands are directed toward each other (Figure 166). Lower your arms and repeat the desired number of repetitions.

3 sets of 20 repetitions

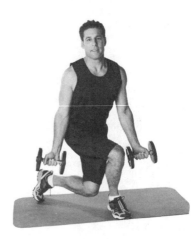

Figure 165

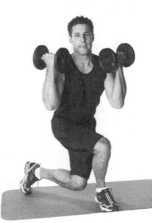

Figure 166

left lunge hold with double row and double triceps kickback (female)

READY: Core, quadriceps, gluteus maximus, hamstrings, calves, inner thighs, triceps, and balance

SET: Stand with a dumbbell in each hand, your palms facing backward. Step forward with your left foot. You can lower your right knee close to the floor to work the legs harder if you choose. Make sure your left knee is directly above your left heel and at a 90-degree angle. Lower your upper torso so that your chest is almost resting on your left thigh and your back is slightly arched.

Remain in this position throughout the exercise.

GO: Lower your arms down to the floor, hands holding the dumbbells with palms facing backward (Figure 167). Bring your arms toward your body in a rowing motion, as high as you can (if you were holding a barbell, it would touch your chest) as you twist your wrists so your palms face each other at the top of the movement (Figure 168).

Then raise your elbows as high as you can, keeping them tight into your rib cage, and using your elbow joint as a hinge, extend the dumbbells backward, leading with the heels of your hands, until your arms are fully extended (Figure 169). Hold for a beat, then unlock your elbows, and release your arms back down to the start position, twisting your wrists at the same time (Figure 167).

3 sets of 20 repetitions

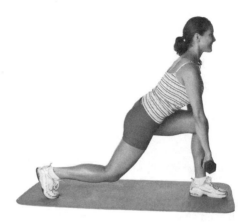

Figure 167

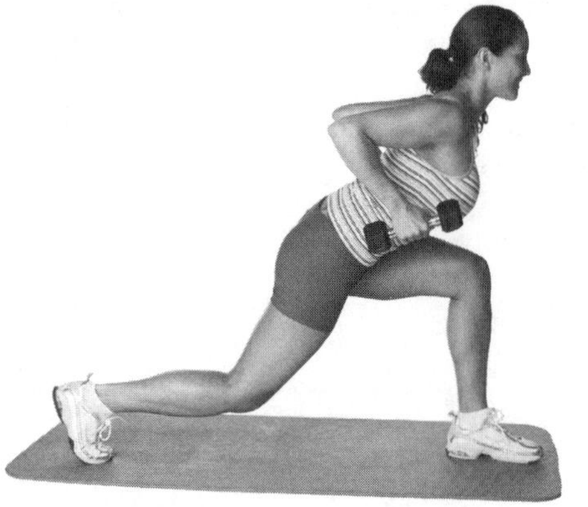

Figure 168

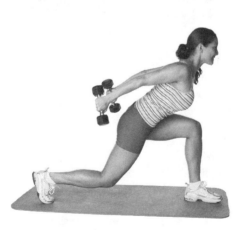

Figure 169

squat and calf raise with double triceps kickback (male)

READY: Core, quadriceps, hamstrings, gluteus maximus, outer thighs, calves, lower back, and triceps

SET: Stand with your feet slightly more than shoulder width apart and your toes turned out slightly, a dumbbell in each hand, your elbows raised as high as possible and held tightly into the rib cage (Figure 170).

GO: Arch your back slightly, keeping your torso over your pelvis. Then lower yourself as if you were sitting in a chair, going down as far as is comfortable.

simultaneously:

Extend your arms backward from the hinge of the elbow (Figure 171). Hold for a beat, then release your arms back to the start position as you raise back up to a standing position. Then jut your hips slightly forward to get a glute contraction and rise up onto your toes in an explosive movement, contracting your calves (Figure 172). Hold for a beat, then release back to the floor.

3 sets of 20 repetitions

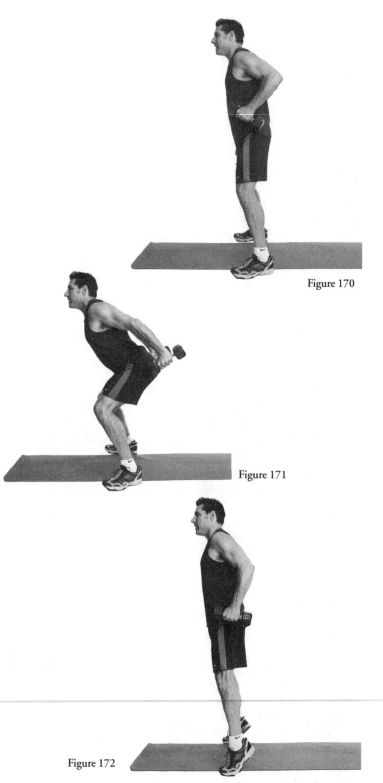

Figure 170

Figure 171

Figure 172

CHAPTER ELEVEN

YIN AND YANG STRETCHING

Up to this point we have discussed in depth Fat-Blasting Nutrition (nutrition plan), Superfast Sculpting (cardio exercise), and 2-in-1 Strength Training (toning). With the knowledge of these three components of your fitness regimen, you should feel extremely confident that you have all the education and information you need to develop your desired body. However, a complete fitness regimen contains not just three but four components. The last component is the one most often overlooked: flexibility or range-of-motion exercise, most often referred to as stretching.

Stretching tends to be overlooked because we don't perceive it as an activity that directly affects our body image or the way our body looks. That is a fallacy. Range-of-motion training is as important as a healthy diet, cardio exercise, and strength training, but for different reasons. Today we live in the most sedentary society ever due to the industrial revolution and modern technology. We sit in a car or a bus on our way to work instead of walking or riding a horse. We sit at the office all day, working on the computer or making phone calls, instead of plowing the fields or spending the day preparing foods from scratch. We sit on the couch at the end of a long day and watch television or play video games instead of finishing our chores for the next day or playing outside with friends. These changes in our society may have improved our ability to accomplish more with less effort, but that is a double-edged sword and has caused other problems.

In addition to the high incidence of obesity, heart disease, and stress-related diseases, our society suffers from an escalated prevalence of chronic joint pain due to lack of motion. More people are suffering from chronic joint pain than ever before, and it stems from acute immobility, musculoskeletal dysfunction, and poor posture. Is it any wonder that 80 percent of our population has experienced back pain? We have become a society in which the cure for almost any pain symptom is a pill. Anti-inflammatory medications such as Celebrex and Vioxx have been prescribed without even a thought about what may be going on with the body structurally. Also, the medications being prescribed for pain or inflammation may not even be safe for you. Vioxx, probably the second-most prescribed anti-inflammatory behind Celebrex, was recently taken off the market because it increased the risk of heart attacks and stroke. What you may not know, however, is that Vioxx was on the market for several years with the manufacturer's knowledge that it was dangerous before it was taken off the market. You can thank the FDA for that. Don't you think a little stretching once in a while may be safer than popping pills? It is not motion but the lack of motion that is the culprit. Every time we move, our body uses a host of muscles to facilitate that movement. If a certain muscle group is shortened, weak, stiff, or tight, the body will hijack peripheral muscles to help complete that movement, which then causes muscle imbalances. Over time the peripheral muscles that are being used to compensate for the weakness of others are compromised. This leads to muscle dysfunction, imbalance, and eventually structural problems. Regular stretching is a way of putting our body into motion that requires minimal effort, prevents and reduces muscle imbalances, helps to prevent injuries, speeds up recovery rates, and, believe it or not, affects our physical appearance.

Structural Problems

How many times have you seen an elderly person with their neck jutted forward, shoulders rounded, and head facing downward? How about someone with rounded shoulders and a little hump on his or her back? This is known as kyphosis, a convex curvature of the spine that stems from tight muscles and tendons and bad posture over a long period of time. I realize that it is hard to imagine ending up like this because you may still be very young (or fairly young) and can still move around quite easily. However, being overweight, walking in high heels, having weak stomach or lower back muscles, and sitting for long periods of time can all lead to poor posture and structural damage. Structural problems develop slowly, over a period of time, without our really even noticing them. Then one day we look in the mirror and notice that our shoulders are a little rounded, our neck or pelvis juts forward, and we have terrible posture. Our body structure has changed over time because our range of motion has been limited. A shortening of muscle tissue, connective tissue, and tendons has occurred, and now our body has a new structure that we don't like. Sitting for long periods of time, for example, whether at your desk, in your car, or at home on the couch shortens your hip flexors, which promotes poor neuromuscular efficiency (the ability of the nervous system to utilize the correct muscles for movement and stability). Sitting also collapses your thoracic region (midback) forcing your shoulders to slump forward, thus placing more stress on your trapezius and lower back. This deficiency will eventually affect motion in the joints and change movement patterns that the body is used to. By the way, this changed pattern causes connective tissue trauma (spasms, knots in soft tissue), which in turn causes inflammation. It's no wonder so many of us have lower back pain and tension in the shoulders. Maybe you have suffered from some structural problem and are experiencing pain. Have you looked in the mirror lately and wished you had better posture? Stretching and range-of-motion exercise can prevent and improve such structural problems. We have been told that to be perceived as self-confident and powerful, we must walk with our head held high, shoulders back, and chest out. People who slouch are perceived as unconfident and lazy. In truth, adding this final fourth component to your new, healthy lifestyle will affect the way your body looks and how people perceive you.

You may know someone who experiences ongoing back pain. How many people do you know who have had back surgery or are on anti-inflammatory or pain medication for back problems? How many of your coworkers are constantly complaining of lower back pain or neck or shoulder stiffness from sitting at a computer all day long? Let me be honest here: chronic pain is not a symptom of being weak or getting older; it is a warning sign of potential danger. It is your body telling you that there is a dysfunction that is being exacerbated by extreme lack of motion. Most people I know sit at a computer for some period of time every day. As I stated earlier, when we sit slumped forward, as many of us do, we experience an increase in thoracic kyphosis (rounded shoulders) and a decrease in lumbar lordosis (concave curvature of the spine), which puts excess stress on the discs of the lumbar spine and increases the compressive force in the wrong areas of the spine. Over time this excess stress and compressive force on the spine will induce mid and lower back pain, as well as neck and shoulder stiffness, and will eventually result in poor posture and some form of pain.

Understanding Musculoskeletal Anatomy

Flexibility is determined by the range of motion in and around each joint. Tight, stiff muscles can limit our normal range of motion and cause musculoskeletal problems, increasing the possibility of soft-tissue injuries. How flexible we are determines how far we can reach, turn, rotate, and bend without tearing or pulling muscles, tendons, or ligaments. Muscle tissue is made up of dense muscle fibers and is connected to the bones by tendons, which are made up of dense connective tissue that is strong and pliable. Ligaments are durable, highly fibrous connective tissues that anchor bone to bone and help protect joints from excess movement. All have the property of elasticity, which refers to their ability to be stretched without tearing. However, as we get older the elasticity in our muscles, tendons, and ligaments declines, which shortens them. Think of a new rubber band. When it's new you can stretch it forever and it won't break. However, after it gets older, it doesn't take much of a stretch to snap it. This is exactly what happens with your muscles, ligaments, and tendons. On the flip side, repeated stretching manipulates the surrounding connective tissue, which, in turn, lengthens muscles, tendons, and ligaments.

When you contract a muscle, you shorten it; when you release or extend a muscle, you lengthen it. We all know how important it is to participate in cardio exercise and resistance training to decrease body fat; increase lean muscle mass; gain strength, power, and endurance; and kick the metabolism into high gear. However, both activities place greater strain on the body and can also shorten muscles, tendons, and ligaments. This is exactly why the fourth and final component of a complete exercise regime is stretching. Tight, stiff muscles disrupt healthy muscle action. If muscles are not able to contract and release properly, there will be a decrease in their performance. This results in less muscle movement and control, causing a loss in strength, power, coordination, and balance.

This is one of the reasons many elderly people have a tendency to fall. Not only are their muscles weak and atrophied, they are stiff due to lack of motion, which inhibits their sense of balance and eye-hand coordination.

Range-of-motion exercise is not something to be taken lightly or viewed as something you will do when you have the time. It is an integral part of a complete exercise regime that directly relates to injury and disease prevention. As we spend more time behind our desks, it is imperative that range-of-motion exercise become a part of our daily routine. Almost every new client who comes to me has some form of structural problem and many times they are completely oblivious to it until I point it out to them. That's because, as I mentioned previously, structural problems develop slowly, over time, and aren't obvious unless pain is involved. However, as a fitness professional who deals with bodies all day long, I can spot problems within seconds of seeing a new client sit or walk. The most prominent dysfunction is what I refer to as collapsed thoracic syndrome. Due to excessive sitting, the thoracic area is collapsed due to midback (thoracic) weakness and reduced range of motion. The lumbar curvature is then compromised by the same issues, causing the rounding of shoulders and slouched posture.

Other typical problems include tight hamstrings (which pull on the lower back) and tight hip flexors (which can cause an anterior tilt of the pelvis and reduce the range of motion of the hip joint). Hip rotation, foot pronation and supination (rotation of the foot), and knee and shoulder misalignment are also very common. These are just a few of the structural issues that can cause serious problems if ignored. I would guess that many people who resort to surgery to correct structural problems could have prevented it had they paid attention to their bodies sooner. More often than not, surgery does not fix the problem. One client who was referred to me by a colleague had suffered from back pain for more than fifteen years. He did not have one day without back pain, and this was after surgery and years of being on pain medication. He had rationalized not exercising by convincing himself that it would only make matters worse. This is often the mind-set of both the medical community and the patient: don't do anything to make it worse. Unfortunately, this is exactly what keeps people in pain; weak structural muscles and lack of motion. Within three months of my working with this client, using a strengthening and stretching routine that was specific to his structural issues, his pain had subsided to just mild, intermittent pain. After six months he was virtually pain-free as long as he adhered to the daily stretching routine we had developed together. I say "we had developed" because everyone's body reacts differently to specific movements and stretches and only the client and his body awareness can determine how a specific exercise or stretch feels. Today, almost two years later, this particular client is pain-free and medication-free and living a healthy lifestyle. He will remain pain-free as long as he adheres to his daily stretching regime and strength trains consistently. If he stops either activity, his body will once again begin to adopt bad habits, and eventually he could begin to experience back pain again. Stretching and range-of-motion exercise can improve, and in many cases eliminate, pain and structural issues if adhered to consistently.

There are numerous other reasons to do flexibility exercises, primarily injury prevention and faster recovery time. By stretching regularly, we reduce the chance of injuring ourselves in normal day-to-day activities. How many times have you turned your head abruptly and ended up with a stiff neck and pain that ran down your back? That might have been prevented with regular stretching of the neck and shoulders. What about the weekend warrior who goes out and plays a game of flag football, pickup basketball, or softball without stretching and ends up pulling a hamstring, straining a groin muscle, or, worse, laid up with a back spasm? When we strain or pull a muscle or tendon, we put a chink in the armor of that particular soft-tissue area. Think of a metal chain: if you stretch the chain, even with extreme force it will not break; however, take a cutter and cut one link, and the next time you place stress on the chain it will snap. Soft-tissue injuries create a weak link in the chain and make your body much more susceptible to injury in the future. Just ask any professional athlete whose career was cut short due to a hamstring, groin, or Achilles tendon tear how painful and debilitating soft-tissue injuries can be. These injuries can be reduced or avoided by taking just a few minutes to stretch before and after participating in any sport or exercise activity. Stretching facilitates body awareness and puts us in touch with areas of our body that may be tight, stiff, or weak so that we can remedy the problem.

In response to excess stress on the muscles, for example in strength training, the body produces lactic acid to protect the body from the large amount of blood that is being pumped into and accumulated in the muscles. This lactic acid in our muscle tissue produces the muscle soreness you feel after a particularly hard exercise session. Stretching after any exercise session will aid the body in releasing the lactic acid from muscle cells faster and more efficiently so that free radicals and other toxins can be quickly removed from the body. This is another reason why warm-up and cool-down periods are important when doing any exercise. The body pumps blood and oxygen to the muscles that are being exercised. At the end of the exercise session, that blood needs to be pumped back to the heart, but there is less force pumping that blood, causing the blood to pool. This causes the onset of muscle soreness. Warming-up ensures that muscle tissue, tendons, and ligaments are properly primed for the added stress because it creates a slow, gradual increase in the circulation of blood. Cooling down allows the body to have additional time to pump blood back to the heart without being under an extreme workload. This reduces blood pooling and the onset of muscle soreness. Stretching on top of cooling down lessens recovery time by reducing muscle soreness and helping the body get rid of waste products faster.

In the Body Express Makeover I have included three stretches that are highly effective in strengthening the thoracic muscles, loosening tight lower back muscles, and improving the lumbar curvature. I have also developed two total-body stretching routines. The first routine is comprised of primarily traditional Western stretches. The second routine is made up of a series of yoga postures meant to stretch and lengthen every muscle group. I have included two stretching routines for variety and to introduce many of you to yoga for the first time. You don't have to do each stretching routine in its entirety every time you stretch, but I would recommend you do the entire routine as often as you can. You can also trade off doing one routine one day and the other routine the next. They both provide flexibility and range-of-motion benefits. After a period of time you can modify the routines to fit the needs of your body. By then you will know which muscle groups require extra stretching time. I recommend holding each stretch for a minimum of thirty seconds to two minutes on average. For some muscle groups, such as the back, hamstrings, and hips, you may want to hold each stretch for as long as three to five minutes. (These stretches are for both men and women.)

three back stretches

lying wall spread

READY: Releases the lower back; helps to drain waste products from the legs; reduces swelling in the feet produced by standing for long periods of time

SET: Sit beside a wall. Make sure your thighs and buttocks are within 6 inches from the wall.

GO: Sit back so that you are lying down and shift your body so that you can lift your legs up onto the wall (Figure 173). Spread your legs into a V shape, trying to keep your buttocks on the floor. You may have to scoot closer to or farther away from the wall to get comfortable. Allow your legs to slide down the wall gradually, without forcing them (Figure 174). Hold this stretch for 3 to 5 minutes.

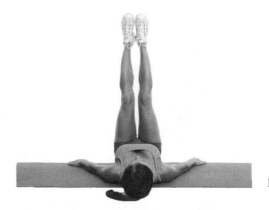

Figure 173

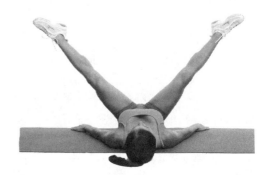

Figure 174

ball superman

READY: Strengthens the thoracic and lumbar areas of the back and glutes.

SET: Kneel with your feet against a wall, a therapy ball in front of you. Drape your torso over the ball, your arms by your sides (Figure 175).

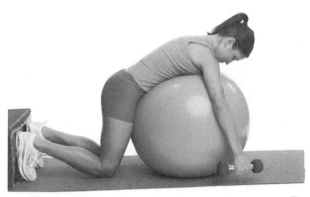

Figure 175

GO: Roll out on top of the ball so that it is under your stomach, your lower back slightly arched, your arms out by your sides, with palms facing your body, your thumbs pointed toward the floor. Your body should be in one straight line. Raise your arms as high as you can squeezing the scapula together and hold the stretch for 20 seconds (Figure 176). Repeat three to five times. For added resistance, you can hold light dumbbells, but remember to keep your thumbs pointed toward the floor (Figure 177).

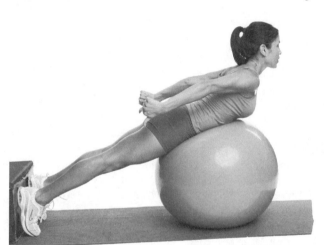

Figure 176

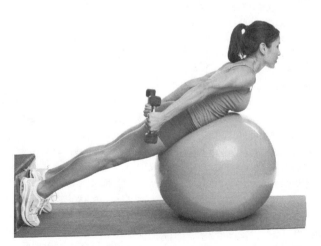

Figure 177

lumbar foam stretch

READY: Reeducates the body about the lumbar curve

SET: Lie on your back with your knees bent.

GO: Lift your hips and slide a small to medium-size foam roller under your lower back. Lower back down, making sure that your buttocks are resting on the floor and the foam roller is directly under your lower back (Figure 178). Wait until your back relaxes and then lower your legs so you are lying on top of the foam roller. (Figure 179). Hold this stretch for 2 to 5 minutes.

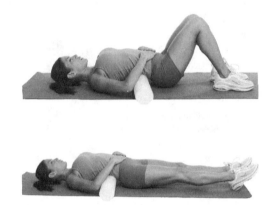

Figure 178

Figure 179

western stretching routine

The Western stretching routine consists of ten stretches that will stretch and lengthen your entire body. You will hold each stretch for a minimum of 30 seconds, up to 2 minutes, on average, depending upon how tight a muscle group is and the specific stretch. You can—and should—hold certain stretches longer than recommended if the particular muscle group affected is tighter than others. The key to lengthening muscle groups is to keep the tension continuous, all the while slowly going deeper into the stretch. Make sure to keep each stretch static, which means no bouncing. Hold the stretch and focus on your breathing. The more normally you breathe, the easier the stretch will be and the greater the benefit you will get from each stretch. So in turn, your focus when doing these stretches should be on your breathing and body awareness. You will begin each stretch with an inhale. Remember to breathe deeply and slowly throughout the routine to allow the body to relax and make each stretch easier. When going deeper into a stretch, always begin with an inhale and then go deeper into the stretch on the exhale.

I recommend that you stretch before and after every cardio and strength training session. I realize that when you have a limited time to work out, stretching is often the component that is skimped on. However, I strongly suggest that you do at least one of the stretching routines in total at least three times per week. If you find yourself pressed for time, stretch for at least 10 minutes prior to exercising and after exercising. Always start out moving into each stretch slowly, especially if you are not warmed up.

The optimal way to utilize each stretching routine would be to warm up for approximately ten minutes with some light cardio activity, then go into one of the stretching routines, which could last from 10 to 15 minutes, depending upon how long you hold each stretch. Then, after you have warmed up and stretched, go into a serious cardio or strength training session. If that's all the time you have for stretching, that's okay; at least you will reduce your chance of injury and increase your overall flexibility. However, if you do have time to repeat one of the stretching routines after your workout, you will begin to change your body structure for the better. The more you stretch the more you will improve your body structure. Now let's get into it.

neck stretch and roll

READY: Stretches and loosens neck muscles

SET: Sit or stand.

GO: Place your right hand on the left side of your head (Figure 180). Slowly pull your head sideways until you feel the stretch (Figure 181). Hold this stretch for 30 seconds to 1 minute, then repeat on the other side. Then roll your neck slowly in a circular motion 4 times in one direction and then 4 times in the opposite direction.

modification: Do not do the neck rolls if you have any cervical injuries.

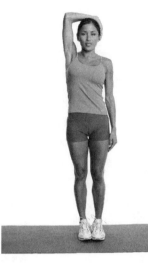

Figure 180

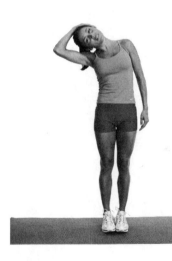

Figure 181

triceps stretch

READY: Stretches the triceps

SET: Sit or stand.

GO: Bring your left arm up and over so that your left hand is on the back of your left shoulder (Figure 182). Take your right hand and place it on top of your left elbow. Slowly pull your left arm back until you feel the stretch in your triceps (Figure 183). Hold this stretch for 30 seconds to 1 minute, then repeat on the other side.

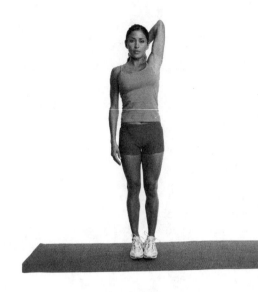

Figure 182

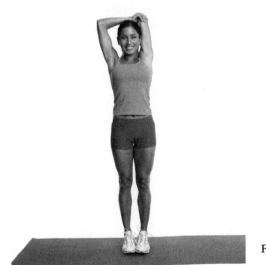

Figure 183

shoulder stretch

READY: Stretches the shoulders

SET: Sit or stand.

GO: Take your right arm across the front of your body, while placing your inside left elbow above your right elbow (Figure 184) and slowly pull your left elbow across your body until you feel the stretch (Figure 185). Hold this stretch for 30 seconds to 1 minute, then repeat on the other side.

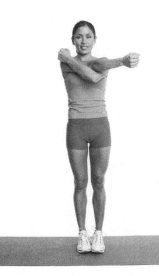

Figure 184

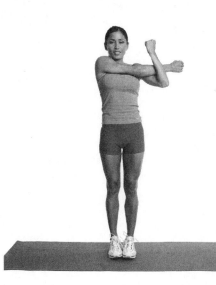

Figure 185

torso stretch

READY: Stretches the entire torso from the waist up

SET: Stand.

GO: Spread your legs wide, your toes facing forward. Pivot your left foot to the side. Slide your right arm down the side of your right leg as you move your left arm up and over to the left side of your body (Figure 186). Keeping your left arm straight and your pelvis in alignment with your body, slowly reach until you feel the stretch (Figure 187). Hold this stretch for 30 seconds to 1 minute, then repeat on the other side.

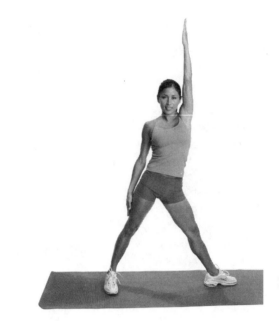

Figure 186

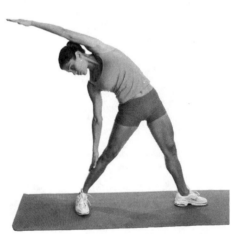

Figure 187

lower back and shoulder stretch

READY: Stretches the lower back, hamstrings, and shoulders

SET: Standing, spread your legs wide, your knees slightly bent, toes facing forward. Bring your arms behind you, clasping your hands together (Figure 188).

GO: Slowly bend forward at the waist, at the same time raising your arms upward, until you feel the stretch (Figure 189). Hold this stretch for 30 seconds to 1 minute, then repeat.

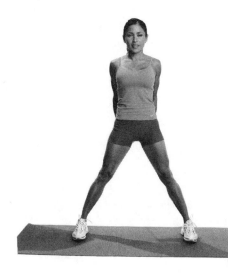

Figure 188

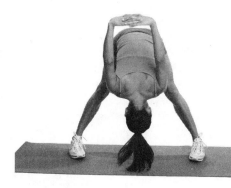

Figure 189

lunge hold

READY: Stretches the groin muscle, hip flexors, hamstrings, calves, and quadriceps

SET: Stand with your hands by your sides (Figure 190).

GO: Step out with your left leg so you are in a lunge position. Keep your back straight by placing both hands on your left leg for stability and pushing your upper torso backward, while pushing back with your right heel (Figure 191).

modification: Place your right knee on the ground and jut your left leg forward (Figure 192).

Hold this stretch for 30 seconds to 1 minute, then repeat on the other side.

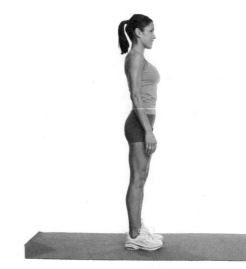

Figure 190

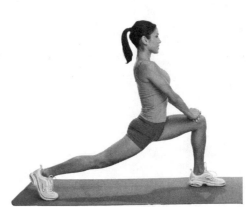

Figure 191

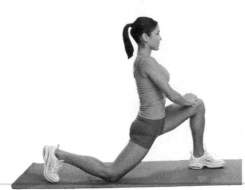

Figure 192

knees into chest

READY: Stretches the lower back and hamstrings

SET: Lie down with your legs bent and your feet on the floor (Figure 193).

GO: Bring both legs up toward your chest, while wrapping your arms around both knees and clasping your hands together (Figure 194). Hold this stretch for 30 seconds to 1 minute, then lower your right leg to the floor and wrap both hands around your left leg (Figure 195). Hold this stretch for 30 seconds to 1 minute, then repeat with the other leg.

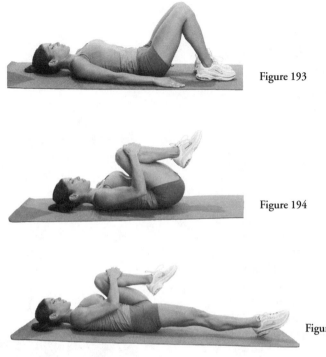

Figure 193

Figure 194

Figure 195

hamstrings/calves/ lower back combination stretch

READY: Stretches the hamstrings, calves, lower back, and hips

SET: Lie down with your legs bent and your feet on the floor (Figure 196).

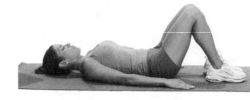

Figure 196

GO: Wrap a towel around the *middle* of your left foot and bring your straight or slightly bent left leg up toward the ceiling while holding on to both ends of the towel until you feel the stretch in your hamstring (Figure 197). Apply continuous tension so that your left leg gradually goes back further throughout the stretch. Hold this stretch for 1 to 2 minutes, then repeat with the right leg.

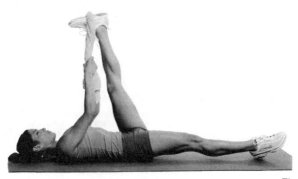

Figure 197

Then wrap the towel around the *top* of your left foot and bring your slightly bent left leg up toward the ceiling while holding on to both ends of the towel until you feel the stretch in your calf. Apply continuous tension so that your left calf gradually goes back further throughout the stretch (Figure 198). Hold this stretch for 1 to 2 minutes, then repeat with the right leg.

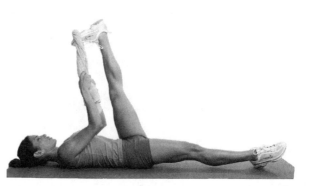

Figure 198

Then drop the towel and lay your left leg across your body, keeping both shoulders flat on the floor, your left arm flat on the floor with the elbow bent at a 90-degree angle (Figure 199). With your right hand, pull your left leg down until you feel the stretch. Hold this stretch for 1 to 2 minutes, then repeat with the right leg.

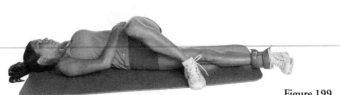

Figure 199

lower back arch

READY: Stretches the upper torso and abdominals and engages the lower back

SET: Lie down on your stomach. Place both hands on the ground under your shoulders, shoulder width apart (Figure 200).

GO: Arch your body upward by extending your arms, keeping your pelvis on the floor, until you feel the stretch (Figure 201).

modification: If you have lower back problems, you can do this stretch resting on your elbows instead of your hands or arch up only as far as is comfortable.

Hold this stretch for 1 to 2 minutes.

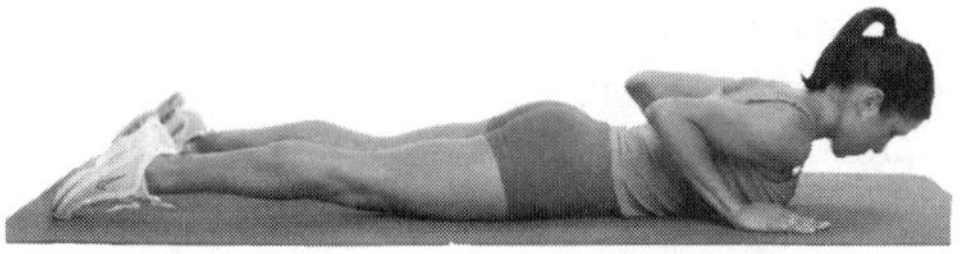

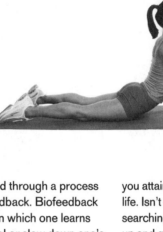

Figure 200

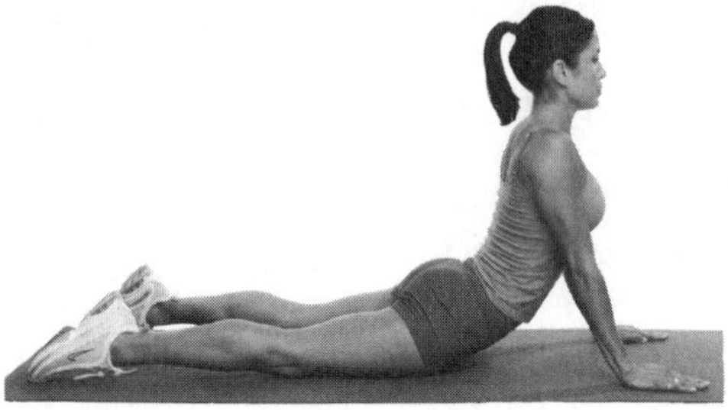

Figure 201

yoga stretching routine

Yoga was developed in India well over five thousand years ago as a means of preparing the body for meditation practice and as a tool to connect the mind and body to facilitate a higher level of awareness. Because meditation involves sitting for long periods of time, which makes the body stiff, yoga was a tool that helped open up the body's energy channels so that energy (*chi*) could flow freely throughout the entire body. Energy continually flows through the body, and the type of energy that flows through yours determines whether you feel scattered, or focused and calm. Getting in touch with your own energy system re-

laxes the mind through a process called biofeedback. Biofeedback is a method in which one learns how to control or slow down one's voluntary (muscle tension) or involuntary (heart rate, circulatory system, blood pressure) physiological responses.

I am an avid practitioner of yoga and consider it to be a physical form of meditation in and of itself. The practice of yoga often slows down the mind, reducing daily stress and the chatter that goes on in our heads all day long. We have thousands of thoughts every day that force us to react in some form without our even being conscious of it. This is the cause of stress, which is the instigator of numerous adult-onset diseases (among them cancer and heart disease). Practicing yoga postures will not only lengthen your muscles, tendons, and ligaments, it will also reduce stress and, in doing so, help

you attain more balance in your life. Isn't that what we are all searching for? To be able to wake up and go through our day with an overall sense of peace and calm, no longer reacting to every single thing that is said or done to us. Balance in life is freedom from the illusion that life needs to be difficult. Life does not have to be a daily battle; it can be a life in which each day provides a new set of challenges, joys, and loving moments.

When doing this yoga stretching routine, you will want to approach the various postures from a place of surrender. In other words, allow your body to relax into each pose, as opposed to pushing deeper into poses before it's ready. The important thing is not to do each pose perfectly but to allow your body to progress into doing each pose as best you can in any given moment. Always breathe through your nose while doing each posture. Inhale before you begin a posture, and exhale as you move into it. Notice how relaxed you are after doing the yoga stretching routine, and try to keep this state of mind throughout your day. Being in a relaxed state of mind encourages being present in the moment, which allows us to experience life to the fullest.

standing side stretch

READY: Stretches the upper torso and obliques

SET: Stand with your feet together and your toes facing forward (Figure 202).

GO: Keeping your right arm straight, bring it up and out to the side of your body until it is next to your ear (Figure 203). Inhale and slide your left arm down the side of your left thigh as you move your right arm up and over to the left side of your body. Keep your right arm straight, your fingers spread, the palm facing down; looking forward, and with your pelvis in alignment with your body, slowly reach until you feel the stretch. Extend this stretch on the exhale (Figure 204). Hold this stretch for 30 seconds to 1 minute or 5 to 10 breaths, then repeat on the other side.

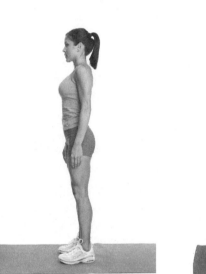

Figure 202

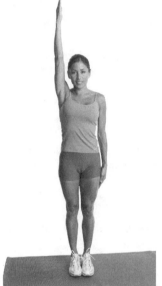

Figure 203

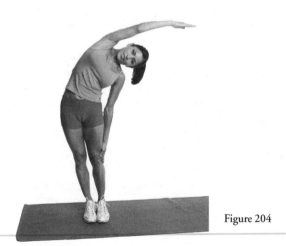

Figure 204

chair pose

READY: Stretches the abdominals and shoulders, opens chest, and engages lower back

SET: Stand with your feet together and your toes facing forward (Figure 205).

GO: Inhale and reach upward from the shoulders, keeping your elbows straight, both palms coming together at the top (Figure 206). Bend your knees and arch your back (Figure 207). Hold this stretch for 30 seconds to 1 minute or 5 to 10 breaths, then repeat. When coming back up to the standing position, exhale and release your arms back to your sides.

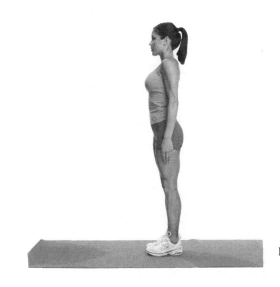

Figure 205

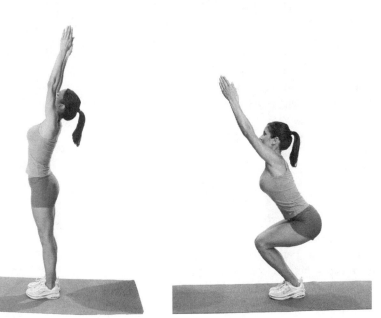

Figure 206

Figure 207

standing forward bend

READY: Stretches the spine, lower back, and hamstrings while relieving tension in the lower back and the entire body

SET: Stand with your feet together and your toes facing forward (Figure 208).

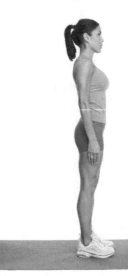

Figure 208

GO: Inhale and bring your arms out to the side and then overhead, palms together (Figure 209). Exhale as you slowly fold forward from your hips and bring your arms out to the sides and then down toward the floor, wrapping your arms around the back of your legs, keeping your legs straight but not locked; push your buttocks upward, elongating your spine until you feel the stretch (Figure 210). Hold this stretch for 30 seconds to 1 minute or 5 to 10 breaths.

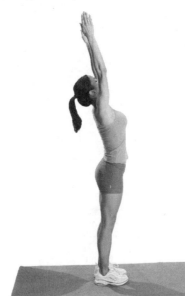

Figure 209

modification: Don't force yourself to go down farther than your body allows. You can use a yoga brick to put your hands on for support if you cannot reach the floor.

When coming back up, inhale and raise your body upward, keeping your spine elongated while bringing your arms out to your sides and then overhead when you reach the standing position.

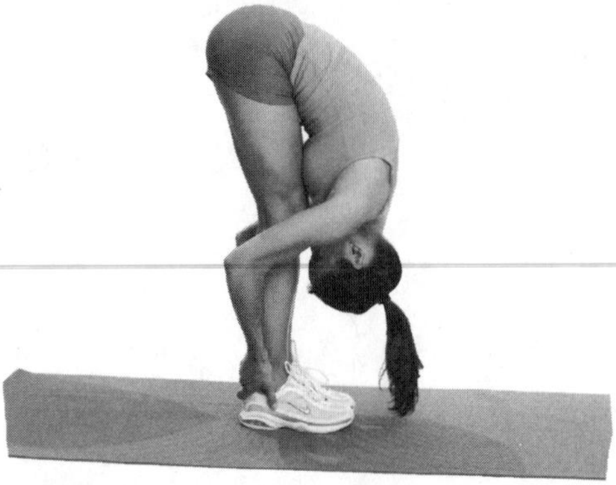

Figure 210

Then spread your legs wide, clasping your hands behind you. Inhale, lengthen your spine, exhale, and fold forward from your hips, raising your arms up behind you (Figures 211 and 212). Hold this stretch for 30 seconds to 1 minute or 5 to 10 breaths.

modification: Don't force yourself to go down farther then your body allows.

When coming back up, inhale and raise your body upward, keeping your spine elongated while bringing your hands back to your sides.

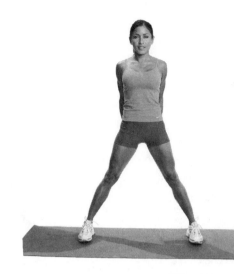

Figure 211

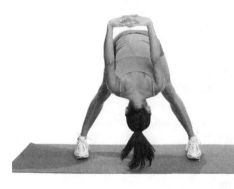

Figure 212

downward dog

READY: Stretches the entire body—primarily the hamstrings, calves, and shoulders—and relieves shoulder and mid back tension.

SET: Get down on your hands and knees (Figure 213). You can also start this pose from the standing forward bend (page 182).

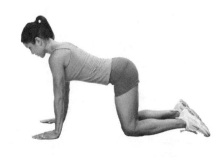

Figure 213

GO: With your hands under your shoulders, lift your knees off the ground, and raise your hips, while turning your toes under so that your feet are flat on the ground. Continue to lift your hips, while pressing your heels and calves into the floor (Figure 214). The key in this pose is to keep pushing backward from your shoulders so that your back is straight and your hips are pushing upward.

modification: Don't force yourself to go back farther than your body wants to.

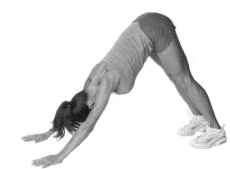

Figure 214

Hold this stretch for 30 seconds to 1 minute, or 5 to 10 breaths. Exhale and go back down on all fours. Repeat.

crescent pose

READY: Stretches the groin, hip flexors, hamstrings, calves, and quadriceps, and improves balance

SET: Stand with your arms by your sides. You can also start this pose from Downward Dog (page 184).

GO: Step out with your left leg while turning your right foot outward, making sure that your right heel is in alignment with your left heel (Figure 215). Slowly bend your left knee, keeping your right leg straight. Inhale, lifting your arms out to the sides and over your head, palms facing inward. Focus on opening your hips by adjusting your left leg outward while keeping your right hip opening in the opposite direction (Figure 216).

modification: Don't force yourself to go farther down than your body wants to.

Hold this stretch for 30 seconds to 1 minute or 5 to 10 breaths. Inhale and straighten your left leg, release your arms back to your sides, and return to the standing position. Repeat on the other side.

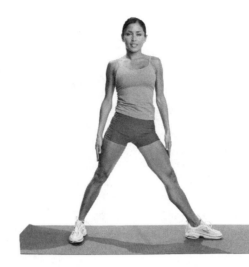

Figure 215

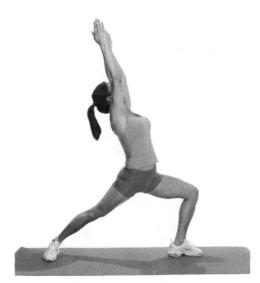

Figure 216

prayer twist

READY: Stretches the spine and lower back, groin, hip flexors, hamstrings, and calves, and improves balance

SET: Stand with your arms by your sides (Figure 217). You can also start this pose from the Crescent Pose (page 185).

GO: Inhale. Then exhale and step out with your right leg so you are in a lunge position (Figure 218). Twist your torso from the hips, moving your left elbow past the outside of your right knee and placing it on your right thigh as your hands move into a prayer position. Push your left elbow into your right thigh as you push your right elbow upward while looking upward until you feel the stretch in your spine and lower back (Figure 219).

modification: You can do this pose with your back knee on the floor.

Hold this stretch for 30 seconds to 1 minute or 5 to 10 breaths. Exhale and straighten your left leg, release your arms back to your sides, and return to the standing position. Repeat on the other side.

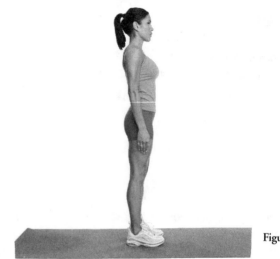

Figure 217

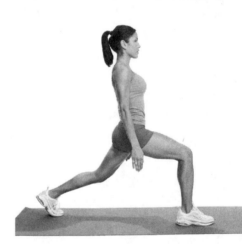

Figure 218

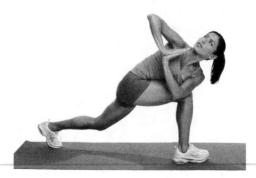

Figure 219

triangle pose

READY: Stretches the torso, shoulders, groin, hip flexors, hamstrings, and calves, and improves balance

SET: Stand with your arms by your sides. You can also start this pose from the Crescent Pose (page 185) or Prayer Twist (page 186).

GO: Inhale. Then step out with your left leg and pivot your right foot inward at a 45-degree angle so that your heels are in alignment and your weight is distributed evenly (Figure 220). Exhale again and lengthen your spine as you lower your left arm to the floor on top of your left foot while raising your right arm straight upward (Figure 221). Stretch your right arm over your ear with your palm facing downward (Figure 222).

modification: If going down to the floor is too difficult, lower your hand as far as you comfortably can and place it on top of your right leg. Extend on the exhale.

Hold this stretch for 30 seconds to 1 minute or 5 to 10 breaths. Exhale slowly and return to the standing position with your hands by your sides. Repeat on the other side.

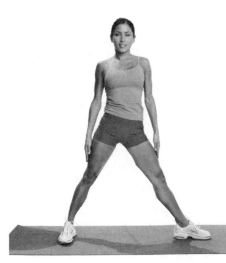

Figure 220

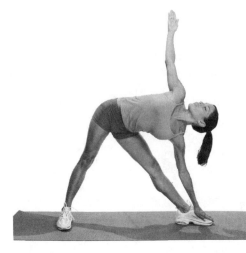

Figure 221

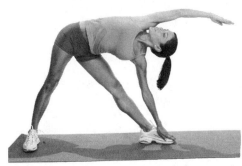

Figure 222

upward dog

READY: Stretches the entire front of the torso, abdominals, shoulders, lower back, and hip flexors, while engaging the glutes and opening up the chest so you can breathe more deeply; also helps to improve posture by pushing the shoulders back and engaging the lower back

SET: Stand with your arms by your sides. You can also start this pose from the Triangle Pose (page 187), Prayer Twist (page 186), or Downward Dog (page 184), or lying on the floor (Figure 223).

GO: Inhale. Then exhale and step or jump back with both feet so that you are now in a plank or push-up position (Figure 224). Inhale and lower your hips, moving your torso forward while rolling over the top of your toes so that your toes are on the floor pointing backward. Pull your shoulders back, raising your chest and your thighs off the ground (Figure 225).

modification: You can do this pose with your thighs on the ground (Figure 226). You can also begin by lying on the floor, pushing up only as far as feels comfortable.

Hold this stretch for 30 seconds to 1 minute, or 5 to 10 breaths. Exhale and slowly lower your knees to the floor. Push backward so that you are resting on your hands and knees or simply lie on the floor in preparation for the next pose.

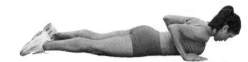

Figure 223

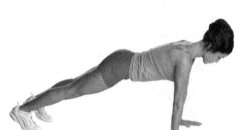

Figure 224

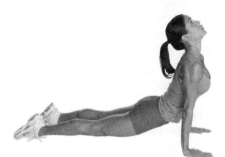

Figure 225

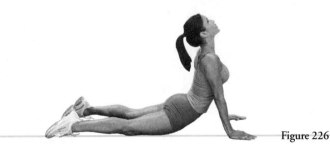

Figure 226

cobra

READY: Stretches the entire front of your torso, abdominals, and lower back while engaging the glutes and opening the chest so you can breathe more deeply; also helps to strengthen the upper back and improve posture by engaging the lower back

SET: Lie down with your thighs together (Figure 227). You can also start this pose from any of the previous postures or from standing.

GO: Place your hands directly under your shoulders with your hands in line with your shoulders. Inhale and arch up, pressing your hips into the floor, while pulling your shoulder blades back to open the chest. Engage your abdominal muscles while pressing your feet into the floor, pulling your shoulders back, and raising your chest upward (Figure 228).

modification: You can rise up only as high as feels comfortable.

Hold this stretch for 30 seconds to 1 minute, or 5 to 10 breaths. Exhale and release your torso to the floor by bending at the elbows.

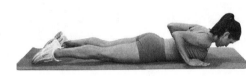

Figure 227

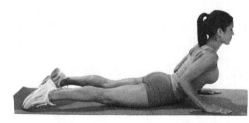

Figure 228

pigeon

READY: Excellent for opening the hips and stretching the periformis muscle, hips, glutes, and thighs; a great stretch for runners or athletes in general who typically get tight hips and periformis muscles

SET: Lie on your stomach. You can also start this pose from Downward Dog (page 184), Upward Dog (page 188), or Cobra (page 189).

GO: From a seated position, place your left leg at a 45-degree angle on the mat in front of you. Lower your upper body on top of your leg so that your left heel is directly under your right hip bone and you are resting on your elbows (Figure 229). If you are very tight in the hips, your left leg will start creeping down to the bottom of the mat as you lie on top of your leg. That is okay. Pigeon is a very intense hip stretch, so work at your own comfort level. If you want to make the stretch deeper, extend your arms in front of you (Figure 230).

modification: If you have bad knees or are extremely tight in the hips, a good modification would be to sit on a mat with your back straight, your left leg behind you, and your right leg out in front of you, slightly bent, with the outside of your foot resting on the mat (Figure 231). Slowly creep your arms forward on both sides of your body, keeping your back straight until you feel the stretch (Figure 232). Work at your own comfort level.

Hold this stretch for 30 seconds to 1 minute or 5 to 10 breaths. Exhale and release your torso

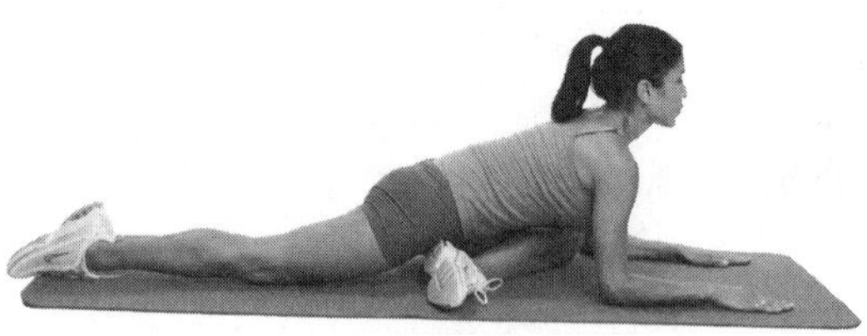

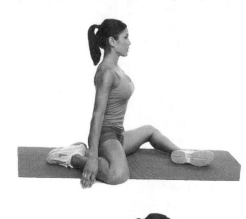

Figure 229

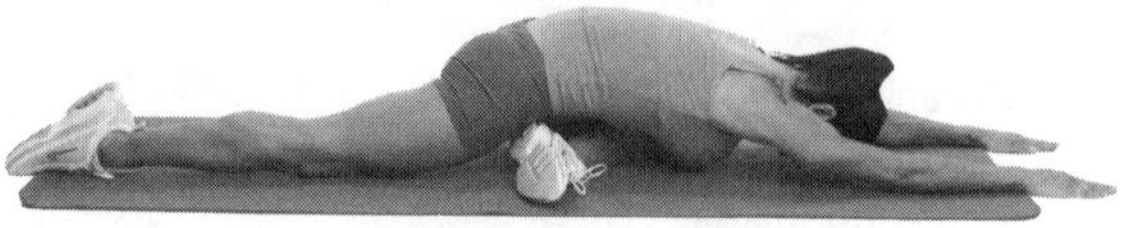

Figure 230

Figure 231

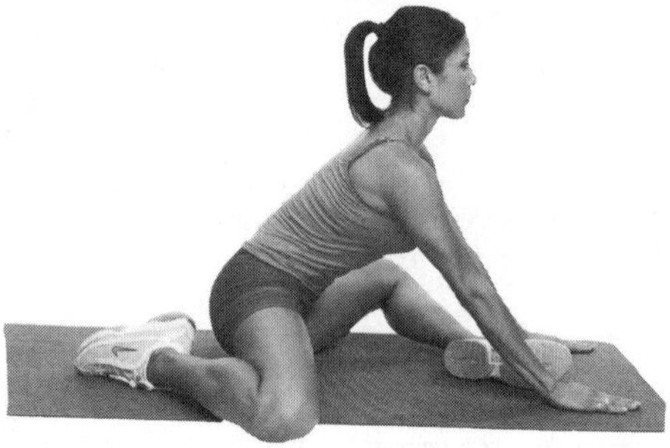

Figure 232

back to sitting, bringing both legs out in front of you, and cross them so you are sitting Indian-style. Remain this way for a moment to access your state of mind.

You may also lie back on the floor into the Shivasana (meditation) Pose with your palms beside your body, facing upward, close your eyes, and just breathe for 3 to 5 minutes. This is a relaxation pose

that will allow you to feel the release of tension and to fully experience the yoga postures you have just completed. Allow your mind to release, free of thought. Let your body melt into the floor. In this pose it is important to do nothing except breathe. In time and with practice, this pose will provide you with the most relaxed state of mind you will ever experience.

CHAPTER TWELVE

MAINTENANCE

Maintenance is the final phase of your body and lifestyle transformation. This is where everything comes together. This is where you have achieved all your goals and reached the final phase of your quest to realize your dream body. You will have altered your lifestyle to support consistent exercise and

healthful eating. You will have learned a lot about yourself during this journey and will have bettered your relationship with yourself as well as with your family and friends. When you arrive at this stage, your life will have been completely altered for the better and for the rest of your life.

When you reach the maintenance stage, I urge you to stop for a moment and congratulate yourself for following through with achieving your dream body and your dream lifestyle. This is a monumental achievement that is worth acknowledging. Don't just pat yourself on the back and continue with your day; take the time to really take in this moment and remember all the time and hard work you have put into the effort. Read through your Notes-to-Self section in your journal and take in the journey you have completed. Many of us tend to be perfectionists and very critical of ourselves, and we never really stop to acknowledge our achievements. We really do ourselves a great disservice when we don't congratulate ourselves or acknowledge how proud we are for fulfilling a commitment. That's a disservice because the human mind

tends to forget very quickly how much work was required to achieve this goal. This is self-defeating and one of the reasons why many people continue on the weight gain, weight loss roller-coaster ride. Use your journal here and write down how you feel about yourself for successfully achieving your goal.

Forgetting how much effort you put into achieving your dream body can cause an unconscious slip into a relapse of weight gain eating and exercising behavior without your really even noticing it until it's too late. As you know, it starts slowly. A pound here, two pounds there, and before you know it you've gained back ten pounds. I call this the negative success syndrome. Sometimes we get so caught up in the fact that we have achieved our weight goal that we get a bit cocky. We start to rationalize that it wasn't that hard to lose the weight and that we will never gain the weight back. I have some unfortunate news for you: if you don't eat healthfully 90 percent of the time and exercise consistently, you will gain the weight back—and fast! Muscle tissue starts to atrophy after 72 hours without strength training exercise. To the human eye it is unnoticeable, but in a few short weeks the lack of muscle tone and strength will be very noticeable.

This brings me to what you will need to do during the maintenance phase. You have achieved your dream body in record time, but in order to maintain that body you will still need to continue with the Fat-Blasting Nutrition strategy, the Superfast Sculpting and the 2-in-1 Strength Training routines consistently. The difference is that you won't have to put in as much time doing your cardio exercise or your 2-in-1 routines. I recommend that you refer back to the cardio chart on page 75 and look at the "Improve heart health" section for your age range and fitness level to determine how much cardio exercise you will need to do each week. Most likely you will probably do twenty to thirty minutes of moderate cardio exercise three to five times per week to maintain your current weight and fitness condition. Of course, you can always do more if you feel the desire. As for the 2-in-1 exercises, I would advise you to refer back to the 2-in-1 chart on page 83 to determine how many of which routines you should do per week. In both areas you want to follow the intermediate guidelines. You will probably do one or more of the 10-, 20-, or 30-minute routines three to five times per week. I would suggest doing no fewer than two 10 Routines and two 20 Routines per week. I encourage all of you to strive to include one 30 Routine in your weekly schedule and to master that very challenging routine.

Don't forget everything you've learned from this book. Use your calendar to schedule all your workouts and meals. Use your journal to help motivate you on days when you just don't feel like exercising. Use the reward system to keep yourself accountable. You are welcome to tailor the reward system however you like, but you should give yourself small intermittent rewards with one large reward at least every three months. If you continue to utilize these motivational and accountability tools, you will maintain your current dream body and reduce any chance of future weight gain or loss of strength or tone. Don't forget to log on to www.body expressmakeover.com every so often for support and encouragement and to provide support for others. "The more you give, the more you get" is a good motto to live by.

Remember to be in the moment and enjoy eating healthfully and exercising consistently as a lifestyle and a journey you will continue for life. Exercising just for body image is a setup for failure because you will never have a perfect body, and even if you did it would never be perfect enough, which would mean that you would always be chasing the elusive carrot.

I too have enjoyed the process of providing you with the knowledge, motivational tools, and guidance to achieve your dream body and dream lifestyle. My passion in life is to help as many people as I can achieve healthy lifestyle transformation, and writing this book has provided me with one more avenue to do so. I encourage you to share this book with friends and family so they too can reap the rewards of a healthier body and a healthier lifestyle. God bless.

REFERENCE LIST

Agatston, M.D., Arthur. *The South Beach Diet.* Emmaus, PA: Rodale, 2003.

Birch, Beryl Bender. *Beyond Power Yoga: 8 Levels of Practice for Body and Soul.* New York: Fireside, 2000.

Clark, Michael A., et al. *Certified Personal Trainer: Optimum Performance Training for the Health and Fitness Professional,* 2nd ed. Calabasas, CA: National Academy of Sports Medicine, 2004.

Deason, Suzanne. *Yoga Conditioning for Weight Loss.* Emmaus, PA: Rodale, 2003.

Egoscue, Pete, with Roger Gittines. *Pain Free: A Revolutionary Method for Stopping Chronic Pain.* New York: Bantam Books, 2000.

Griscom, Chris. *The Healing of Emotion: Awakening the Fearless Self.* New York: Fireside, 1990.

National Strength and Conditioning Association. *Essentials of Strength Training and Conditioning,* 2nd ed. Edited by Thomas R. Baechle and Roger W. Earle. Champaign, IL: Human Kinetics, 2000.

Pilzer, Paul Zane. *The Wellness Revolution: How to Make a Fortune in the Next Trillion Dollar Industry.* Hoboken, N.J.: John Wiley & Sons, 2003.

Prochaska, James O., John C. Norcross, and Carlo C. Diclemente. *Changing for Good.* New York: Avon Books, 1995.

Schiffmann, Erich. *Yoga: The Spirit and Practice of Moving into Stillness.* New York: Pocket Books, 1996.

Schlosser, Eric. *Fast Food Nation: The Dark Side of the All-American Meal.* New York: Perennial, 2002.

Sears, Barry. *A Week in the Zone.* New York: Regan Books, 2000.

———, with Bill Lawren. *Enter the Zone: A Dietary Road Map.* New York: Regan Books, 1995.

Tolle, Eckhart. *The Power of Now: A Guide to Spiritual Enlightenment.* Vancouver, British Columbia: Namaste Publishing, 1999.

INDEX